HAIR COLORING
A Hands-On Approach

HAIR COLORING

A Hands-On Approach

Patricia Spencer
Associate Professor of Cosmetology
Riverside Community College
Riverside, California

Milady Publishing Company
(A Division Of Delmar Publishers Inc.)
3 Columbia Circle, PO Box 15015
Albany, New York 12212-5015

Library of Congress Cataloging-in-Publication Data
Spencer, Patricia
    Hair Coloring: A Hands-On Approach / Patricia Spencer.
      p.   cm.
    Includes bibliographical references and index.
    ISBN 0-87350-393-7
    1. Hair—Dyeing and bleaching.   I. Title.
TT973.S64 1991   90-13380
646.7'242—dc20   CIP

Editors: Catherine Frangie
             Joseph Miranda

Production: John Mickelbank
               Jose Medina
               Lisa Mauro
               John Fornieri
               Barbara Cardillo

Text Design: Arthur Hamparian

Cover Design: Ronald Ridgeway Incorporated

Illustrations: Shiz Horii

Photographs courtesy of: Clairol Inc.
                             Redken Laboratories, Inc.
                             Steven Landis
                             Eric Von Lockhart

Copyright © 1990
Milady Publishing Company
(A Division of Delmar Publishers Inc.)

Printed in the United States of America

10 9 8 7 6 5 4 3

Contents

3—*Semipermanent Hair Coloring* *39*

Preface

The discovery method leads students into the higher levels of learning, past the simple process of recall and application into the uncharted territories of synthesis and evaluation. Heuristic learning challenges students to think logically, analyze a situation, and transfer information from one area to another in order to discover the "truth."

Experiential learning situations, such as those created in this text, painlessly lead students through the highest forms of learning. Students are called upon to involve themselves in a project and to use the elements of synthesis to organize new ideas.

The classroom becomes energy charged. You can *see* learning take place. The experimental learning designed in this text utilizes four of the five senses (no tasting, please). Therefore, the learning is more meaningful and longer lasting. Every experiment takes on a life of its own with unique characteristics. The students learn not only from their lab experiments, but also from the experiences of their classmates.

The students' progress through the cognitive levels of *Bloom's Taxonomy of Thinking*, reaching the evaluation stage. Decisions and judgments must be made based on scientific criteria and industry standards. The finished product of chemical data and completed swatches becomes a complete reference manual for use in any progressive salon.

A survey of cosmetology students, stylists, managers, and salon owners reveals that a lack of expertise in hair coloring is a major concern in our industry. This fact can be financially devastating as hair coloring can easily become the number one money-maker in any salon! The purpose of this book is to emphasize the scientific background in chemistry and physics for those who strive to become expert hair colorists.

The educational experience, as provided by this text, plays another crucial part in our industry. Cosmetology is now classified by the Federal Government as a field utilizing hazardous chemicals and has designated cosmetologists as *chemical workers*. This classification brings with it new safety and educational regulations. The Federal Government, state agencies, and consumer advocate groups have created a mandate for greater understanding of chemistry and increased distribution of scientific data on hair coloring products.

With this mandate comes a legal and moral obligation that the professional cosmetologist cannot ignore. According to a CBS news report, "During one year alone, more than 4,000 Americans were treated in hospital emergency rooms for medical problems caused by hair coloring products." The Chemical Workers Union has created a division to deal with the safety of cosmetologists and barbers. They have issued reports on the safety and legal obligations of cosmetologists who deal with chemicals. Many pending lawsuits directly relate to cosmetologists' ignorance of the products they are using.

Statistics such as these have created legislation that now places responsibility with cosmetologists to educate themselves in an effort to curtail such incidents. It is now the responsibility of salon owners, managers, cosmetology instructors, product distributors, and manufacturers to provide up-to-date information on the safety and chemistry of current technology. One of the goals of this book is to help cosmetologists achieve this level of professionalism.

Most available hair coloring books are written or sponsored by product manufacturers. They offer the colorist only a very limited view of the wide world of color. These books tend to advertise and promote the use of their own product exclusively, to the exclusion of all others, with little or no basis in the science of hair coloring.

Hair Coloring: A Hands-On Approach presents scientific data and controlled experimentation that can be used with any manufacturer's line by all students, schools, and professionals involved in the field of cosmetology. In this field of ours, art and science walk hand in hand. This book can help you achieve a more professional level by providing a secure foundation in physics and chemistry that will allow you to free your natural artistic ability.

A Note to Instructors

Technology is advancing at such a pace as to cause a constant influx of new chemicals, safety data, and coloring products. Continuing education is a must for today's hair colorists. Recently a Federal law was passed that affects cosmetologists as workers in the chemical industry. This law places additional responsibility for the safe use and knowledge of the chemicals used in the formulation of our products.

Hair Coloring: A Hands-On Approach will provide researched scientific chemical and safety data on each classification of hair color accompanied by controlled lab experiments designed to address new health and safety standards and educational codes within the cosmetology industry.

This book is to be used in conjunction with the hair coloring curriculum of all cosmetology programs including beginning, advanced, teacher training, instructor credential, and return to industry courses. It guides any level student through exploration of the true form of hair coloring—an equal blend of art and science. This learning tool will accompany the student colorist into the industry and always remain a useful reference of scientific data and product results.

This book is designed to expand analytical thinking skills. The controlled lab experiments offer the educational experience of analyzing, formulating, documenting, and evaluating the result of applying color on hair swatches before client contact. These activities have been student tested and found to greatly increase the performance, confidence, and safety levels of the students as they enter the work force and are expected to perform at industry standards.

The *Review Questions* at the end of each controlled experiment benefit the students in several ways. First, they challenge students to analyze their educational activity, assess their achievement of the lesson's objectives, and draw conclusions as to the success or failure of the chemical process of each experiment. The questions require that the students judge their own performance and suggest alternate solutions to the problems posed in some of the experiments. This step of learning, known as the evaluative stage, is the highest level of learning.

Secondly, these essay questions require that the students utilize and thereby improve their reading comprehension abilities. The questions challenge the students to identify key points as they read.

Thirdly, the essay questions require that the students utilize and thus improve composition writing skills. The culmination of these benefits is to strive toward the national goal of schools in general—*Reading and Writing Across the Curriculum*.

The lab experiments in this book can be used in a structured classroom setting or they can be used independently. They are excellent methods of challenging the gifted student who soars past the majority of the class. This type of independent, yet directed study prevents the sinking into boredom and discontent that naturally occurs when students are not striving forward.

The materials are designed to assist cosmetology instructors in guiding students through a directed study of hair coloring. The book provides the history, uses, and unique characteristics of color with which instructors can create interest and excitement in classroom lectures. The scientific data necessary to implement the experimentation phase of the lesson on each color classification is provided on all aspects of color.

The essay questions can be utilized in several ways, subject to instructor preference. They can be used as quizzes, tests, or stimuli for small group or classroom discussion. They will help students to improve analytical skills, reading comprehension, and writing abilities. The new lecture information, instructional materials, and controlled experimentation lesson plans will assist instructors by providing a method of stimulating the advanced student with extra-credit projects and with review materials for the less advanced student.

This book fills a void in the educational process of cosmetology students caused by the lack of scientific references on the subject of hair coloring. Unlike all other available hair coloring references, the information contained within is not subject to manufacturer bias and propaganda. This book offers theories, facts, and methods that are applicable regardless of product brand name.

Another key concept to consider in the use of this book is that current curriculum reform trends across the nation call for the development of core curriculum at all levels of education. This text integrates the concepts of history, art, and science in a manner that brings the goals of core curriculum to cosmetology.

Acknowledgments

I wish to express my appreciation to Riverside Community College for their support of my professional growth by allowing me a sabbatical to prepare this manuscript.

I also wish to thank those colleagues who encouraged and supported my efforts through their participation in this project. Thank you to all who utilized and tested the experiments in your classrooms and those who proofread various parts of the manuscript. And a special thanks goes to all the students who tested these experiments and offered suggestions that created better learning situations.

My deepest appreciation goes to my family. My heartfelt thanks to my husband and editor-in-chief, Mike Spencer and our son, Jeffrey. Without the support of these two wonderful men, this endeavor would still be a dream floating around in my head. Thank you.

About the Author

Patricia A. Spencer has been involved in the beauty and fashion industry for 25 years. Her career is multi-faceted. She has been a cosmetology instructor for 14 years and is currently serving as Associate Professor of Cosmetology at Riverside Community College in Riverside, California.

Patricia earned an Associate of Arts degree at Riverside Community College, a Bachelor of Science degree from the University of LaVerne, and both a teaching credential and a Master's degree from the University of California at Riverside. Patricia has also been trained as an Instructional Skills Facilitator through a program originating with the British Columbia Ministry of Education. She has taught all phases of cosmetology, including the teacher training program and advanced courses for licensed cosmetologists, as well as serving as competition coach.

Patricia has assisted the public with their beauty needs on a one-to-one basis and in the capacity of manager of several chains of beauty establishments in California and Colorado. As a member of the National Cosmetology Association, she has held the positions of Director and Chairperson of the Riverside Valley Styles Panel. Patricia has organized and promoted beauty and fashion shows as well as cosmetology competitions throughout Southern California.

As past Fashion and Beauty Editor for *Inland Empire* magazine, Patricia wrote a monthly column as well as articles on community activities and professional women. Her articles, covering such topics as professional technology and teaching techniques, have been published in the *National Beauty School Journal*. She currently writes *Good Looks*, a weekly fashion and beauty newspaper column.

Introduction

Early man chose to surround himself with color because he believed that it made things happen. Colors were symbols of power, mysticism, and religion. Prehistoric man colored his skin and hair in ways that offer insight into how he coped with his environment.

Ancient Grecian mythology tells of man using color to banish demons and evil spirits. Cavemen used minerals, insects, and plants to paint their bodies and color their hair to beautify and identify, to attract and intimidate. Much as we use color yet today!

In 27 B.C. the Gauls, who lived in what is now known as France, dyed their hair brilliant red to indicate a particular class, while the Anglo Saxons in England favored bright green, orange, and blue. In later years, Roman law decreed that yellow or blonde hair would be worn by "women of the night," while in modern England, auburn indicates a royal class, an attempt to emulate Queen Elizabeth.

During the 1800's, American men were excellent color clients. Beard and mustache dyeing was available at the barber shop. Silver nitrate and gold chloride were used, but both faded to strange iridescent hues. In 1825, a product called Grecian Water, with a formula of distilled water, silver nitrate, and gum water, was used for darkening the hair. However, it was far from perfect. After several uses, the hair would turn purple!

Until the 1860's man remained restricted to these natural dye forms derived from mollusks (oysters, clams, snails), insects, plants, vegetables, and earth's components. During this time technology did not allow for the creation of more than a few hundred dyes, which were used to color hair, fabrics, cosmetics, and other manmade goods.

Then by chance, in 1859, color creation experienced a breakthrough. A German professor, Wilhelm Hofman of London's Royal College of Chemistry, was researching coal-tar derivatives. A student of Professor Hofman's, William Henry Perkin, was attempting to synthesize quinine. Instead, he ended up with a useless-looking black sludge. Rather than give up and toss it out, the student began to dilute the sludge with alcohol. The resulting solution was purple.

This was just the beginning of a long and illustrious career that even included knighthood for William Henry Perkin. However, most important to cosmetologists was the fact that his discovery led to the creation of more brilliant and more permanent dyes that could be used on fabric and hair alike. The world no longer had to depend upon colors ground from stone, plants, or animal remains.

The 20th century brought the age of commercial dyes compounded from petroleum products. By 1980, 3,000,000 shades of artificial dye had been created and at least 9,000 of them have been marketed. Through the years, the colors have become more brilliant than ever, showing depths and hues never existing before, except in the imagination. Even though we now have colors of exquisite quality and lasting durability, man is not satisfied. The availability of new and exciting dyes continues to grow at the rate of approximately two per week.

The color industry, through science and technology, has taken great strides away from the ancient Grecian use of color to ward off demons and evil spirits. Throughout the 20th century each decade has been marked by its own fashion trend in color. The colors that are popular at a given time serve as indicators of the state of the nation, the mood of the people.

In 1910, trends in both hair color and fashion became bright and free. Women made more dramatic changes in their hair color than they had in a century, threw away their corsets, and bared their knees.

In the 20's, colors again became more subdued and henna was popular as a hair dye. A 1928 issue of *Good Houskeeping* featured an article titled "Shall I Dye My Hair?" The author, a doctor, advised that henna was the only safe way to dye the hair as all other dyes on the market contained toxic chemicals.

Society of the early 1930's looked upon hair color as a product that "nice women" did not use. At least, not publicly. All hair coloring was done secretly at home or in private salon booths. Women would even go as far as to book salon appointments under an assumed name. However, toward the end of the 30's and early 40's women rebelled against this taboo and openly made their hair coloring appointments.

During the 50's, women began to put blonde, red, blue, and silver streaks into their hair with temporary spray-on hair coloring products. Heavy black eye makeup and a vibrant pink lipstick created a total fashion look that was indicative of the mood during this era.

The 60's brought the invention of "shampoo-in-color," which enabled women to shampoo and dye their hair in one step. However, henna once again made the strongest fashion statement, a trend to the natural-look that *Time* magazine labeled as "The Big Fade."

Both the 70's and the 80's were times of revolutionary change in fashion colors. The 80's ended in an age of "Fashion Freedom." The 90's will provide a virtual smorgasbord of options. While availability and economics at one time dictated what colors would be used in fashion, current technology has made it possible to create any color on any medium, whether it be fabric, plastic, cosmetics, or hair. Today, the imagination sets the only limits on what colors will dominate the fashion world.

The scientific data and product experimentation in this book work together, hand in hand, to create an educational background in the chemistry and physics of color. With this background, you will be able to turn your imagination free. No longer will you have worries such as:

- Did I select the correct color classification?
- Did I formulate correctly?
- Are these chemicals compatible?
- Will I achieve the desired color results?
- Will I be able to remove this color?
- Will I be able to do color corrections?
- How do I add warmth without altering my hue?
- Is this chemical safe for my client?

No longer will you be confused and discouraged by the current technology of our industry. Cosmetologists have always appreciated the artistic side of hair coloring and now the need to understand the science has reached full recognition. Upon completion of this book, you will have the expertise to create any fashion statement possible in the world of color. You will be the expert!

HAIR COLORING
A Hands-On Approach

1

Colorimetry

Colorimetry is the process used by professionals to measure and analyze the composition of a color. The human eye can discern the differences between nine to ten million colors of varying hue, level, and saturation. However, as yet, chemists have been able to duplicate only a very small number of these colors. Color specialists have worked in the Borg-Warner Chemical company for over a quarter of a century to create more than 45,000 colors, yet they have a long way to go before they duplicate the colors found in nature.

As an example of the varieties of hues, levels, and saturations within one color, Borg-Warner has manufactured more than 2,000 shades of white. "White is not just a white," a specialist reported. "There is down, balsa, cream, eggshell, whipcream, pearl, lace, wisp, cloud, frost, ash, fog, mist, warm, eggnog, and sand, to name just a few whites."

COLOR MIXING

Colors are mixed in one of two different ways, depending upon the medium used. These two methods are known as *Subtractive Color Mixing* and *Additive Color Mixing*.

Additive Color Mixing

Additive color mixing is also known as "color by addition." It is the method used to mix colored beams of light. Each color can be separated from the spectrum and beamed onto a certain spot. The beaming of one light on top of the other adds one color to the other, creating a new color. Thus the name "Additive Color Mixing" refers to the fact that a new color is created by adding together the light of different wavelengths.

In this additive method of color mixing, the three primaries are beams of red, blue, and green. A mixture of blue and green light creates blue-green. A mixture of red and green light makes yellow. When focused on the same spot, the combination of all visible light rays creates "white" light. *(See Color Plate 1.)*

Color television pictures are created with this additive color mixing process. A color screen has thousands of tiny areas that glow with different beams of the primary colors when charged with electrons. The combining of the primaries in this way creates the wonderful colors seen on television today.

Subtractive Color Mixing

Subtractive color mixing refers to the fact that the more colors in the mixture, the more color is subtracted or absorbed from the white light rather than being reflected and transmitted to the eye. When light strikes each pigment in the object, the pigment absorbs, or subtracts, different wavelengths from the white light. This causes only the hues reflected in common by all the component pigments to be transmitted to the eye. *(See Color Plate 2.)*

The subtractive method of color mixing is also known as "color by subtraction." The subtractive method of color mixing is the method used to mix all other forms of color other than light rays. It is used in the production of inks, paints, plastics, fabrics, cosmetics, and hair colorings. Identifying, mixing, and achieving a desired shade requires a working knowledge of the Three Dimensions of Color and the Artist's Concept of the Laws of Color.

COLOR FROM LIGHT

Without light, color ceases to exist. Outside your window an hour before dawn, the world is dark. At the beginning of dawn, the world begins to become visible. Vague forms become distinguishable, but they are gray. As the sun peaks over the horizon, the world bursts forth in spectacular color. And this phenomenon occurs because *color is light*.

The 17th century scientist, Sir Isaac Newton, discovered that the "white" light from the sun contains all the colors of the world. He proved his theory by allowing a beam of light to pass through a glass prism. The light waves were bent at different angles to create a fan-shaped series of colors.

You can duplicate this experiment yourself or simply closely observe your next rainbow. You will notice that the colors are always arranged in the same order. Red is at the top of the rainbow, followed by orange, yellow, green, blue, with violet at the bottom.

Light is composed of a wide range of wavelengths that behave much like the waves made by a rock thrown into the middle of a pond. When a beam of light passes through a prism, as first demonstrated by Newton, the rays of different wavelengths are bent at different angles. The bending breaks the sunlight into a beautiful band of colors known as the visible spectrum. The visible spectrum contains all the colors of the rainbow. *(See Color Plate 3.)*

It is the movement of these rays of light that create what we visualize as colors. Red is created by the longest and slowest moving wavelength of light. Further down the spectrum, the wavelengths become shorter and quicker moving. The visible effect of this is that the colors progress from red, to orange, yellow, green, blue, and finally to violet. Violet consists of the shortest and fastest wavelengths of light that can be seen by the human eye. *(See Color Plate 4.)*

The color we see is a result of the process of selective absorption controlled by the pigment of an object, and many different types of pigment exist. Melanin is the pigment of human skin and hair. Carotenoids are the pigments of carrots, salmon, lobsters, and autumn leaves. Anthocyanin pigments color red wine, rhubarb, and beetroot. Hemoglobin is the pigment which carries the oxygen in the bloodstream and gives the blood its red color.

Each of these pigments has the ability to selectively absorb and reflect certain wavelengths. The length and speed of these wavelengths creates a certain image on the eye which is sent to the brain for interpretation. In short, the physics of color tells us that there is no such thing as color. Color is simply a reflection or absorption of the varying movements of lightwaves. And as human beings, we have agreed to call this image color and give the different shades different names such as red, blue, and yellow. *(See Color Plate 5.)*

Now, having said that there is no such thing as color, let us continue our indepth study of this phenomenon, this continual movement of lightwaves, that we have agreed to call color!

THE THREE DIMENSIONS OF COLOR

It is through the naming of colors that we learn to describe, classify, and distinguish one from another. The commercial names given by man to different colors, whether they be paint colors such as "winter white" and "cocoa brown" or hair colors such as "silent snow" and "frivolous fawn," are generally attractive, romantic terms. While these names are wonderful sales tools when discussing color with clients, they are inadequate for purposes of formulation and communication among professionals. The professional colorist must be able to identify color in a more scientific manner.

Arranging the colors of the spectrum in a manner that would join science, art, and beauty is a problem that has plagued philosophers, artists, and mathematicians for centuries.

In the 17th century, Isaac Newton first arranged the colors according to their wavelengths. He placed them in a simple circle of hues, joining the red at one end of the spectrum to violet at the other. However, color is not that simple.

Each color has a great range of variations and intermediate shades. Each color can be intense or pale, warm or cool, light or dark, or any combination thereof.

All colors have three dimensions and each of these three dimensions has three technical names. All three names are correct, but they vary depending upon industry use. These three dimensions are:

1. Hue, color, tone
2. Level, depth, value
3. Saturation, intensity, chroma

Hue

Hue is the basic name of a color, and the term is used interchangeably with color by laymen. Hue tells us to which class a particular color belongs: red, yellow, blue-green, etc. This arrangement in an ordered circular sequence makes color relationships become visibly apparent and easy to work with.

This arrangement of hues in an ordered circular sequence creates the "Chromatic Circle" or basic color wheel. While much is gained by the use of this basic color wheel, it is incomplete without consideration of the remaining two characteristics of every hue: *level* and *saturation*.

Level

Any level or degree of depth can be described in terms of lightness or darkness. Colors lighten when mixed with white, darken when mixed with black, and range somewhere in between when mixed with gray. However, because black is the absorption of all hues, and white is the reflection of all hues, as the level of a color is altered the hue itself also undergoes some change.

The human eye can distinguish as many as 150 levels. However, it is impractical to attempt to work with this many levels for hair coloring purposes. The distinction of level in this industry is on a sliding scale of light to dark, broken into 10 separate levels. Light colors are said to have a higher level (lightest blonde—level 10) and darker colors are said to have a lower level (black—level 1).

Saturation

Saturation presumes the existence of hue. It is the distinction in color of a more saturated or less saturated hue, a more intense or less intense color. In short, it is the amount of hue in a color. Red, for instance, can be more vividly or less vividly red. Unlike hue and level, which can be visualized independently of each other, saturation or intensity cannot be visualized except as a variable in a scale in which level is systematically affected.

When increasing the saturation of a hue, more of the concentrated pigment is added to the formulation. This creates more intensity in the color. As the intensity is increased the level also becomes lower or darker. As the saturation is decreased the level becomes higher or lighter. The difference in this level change from the one that occurs with the addition of white, black, or gray is that the hue remains true.

THE ARTIST'S CONCEPT OF THE LAWS OF COLOR

The Laws of Color are those laws in nature that regulate the creation of color. The Artist's Concept of the Laws of Color are those laws that regulate the mixing of dyes and pigments to create other colors. The colorist can create any hue, level, or saturation by implementing these laws through the subtractive method of mixing.

While the Laws of Color are constant, they are subject to interpretation and personal preference. Artists and scientists alike consider them guidelines for combining colors harmoniously, but there are no fixed rules of color harmony because too many factors affect whether certain colors go together.

Hue

The first concept of these laws is that of basic hue. Hues are arranged around the Chromatic Circle or Color Wheel in a manner that shows the relationship among colors. The hues of the Chromatic Circle are divided into four categories: *primary, secondary, tertiary,* and *quaternary colors.*

The *primary colors* are basic or true colors. A primary color cannot be broken down further into any other color. There are three primary colors: *yellow, red,* and *blue.* These colors are completely pure and cannot be mixed through the combination of other colors.

Using watercolors or fingerpaints, place the primary colors on the color Chromatic Circle in their correct positions.

THE CHROMATIC CIRCLE

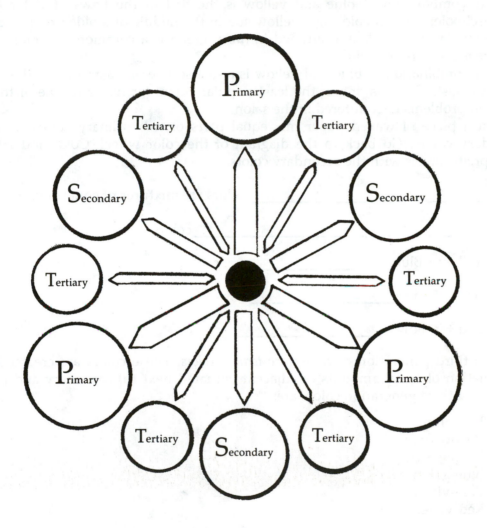

Fill in the Blanks

1. Primary colors are _____ colors.

2. Primary colors _____ be achieved by mixing.

3. The primary colors are _____, _____, and

_____.

The *secondary colors* are the mixture of equal amounts of two different primary colors. For example, mixed in equal parts:

- Yellow + Red = Orange
- Red + Blue = Violet
- Blue + Yellow = Green

Therefore, the three secondary colors are *orange, violet,* and *green*.

The combination of blue and yellow is the first of the Laws of Color learned by preschoolers. When coloring a yellow sun in the middle of a blue sky, it is difficult not to overlap colors. A sun outlined in fuzzy green is a common frustration to the average four-year-old child.

The combination of blue and yellow is also a source of frustration to the average cosmetologist. Green is one of the least popular colors for hair and one of the most common problems encountered in the salon.

On a piece of waxed paper mix equal parts of two primary colors to achieve secondary colors. Go back to the diagram of the color wheel. Color and label the appropriate circles with the secondary colors.

1. _____ colors are mixtures of equal amounts of two

_____ colors.

2. Yellow + Blue = _____ .

Blue + Red = _____ .

Red + Yellow = _____ .

The third generation of colors are *tertiary colors*. These colors are created by the combination of equal amounts of adjacent (situated next to) secondary and primary colors. The third generation colors are:

- Red-orange
- Yellow-orange
- Yellow-green
- Blue-green
- Blue-violet
- Red-violet

On your waxed paper mix equal amounts of one secondary color and an adjacent primary color to achieve the six tertiary colors. Go back to the diagram of the color wheel. Color and label the appropriate circles with the tertiary colors.

1. Tertiary colors are equal amounts of one _____ and one

_____ color.

2. The tertiary colors are _____

_____

The fourth generation of colors are quaternary colors. The quaternary colors are all other combinations that eventually reach all the levels of color that the eye can see.

The Color Triad

Three colors an equal distance apart on the color circle are called a *color triad*. *(See Color Plate 6.)* The colors in a triad, combined in a variety of levels and saturations, generally create a pleasing effect when used together. The primary colors on the Chromatic Circle—red, yellow, and blue—create a triad. The secondary colors—green, orange, and violet—form a triad.

Warm and Cool Hues

As well as being a tool to place the hues as to their relationship, the Chromatic Circle is used to identify the warm and cool hues. To separate the warm from the cool colors, draw a heavy black line from the yellow-green to the red-violet.

Warm hues are those from red-violet to yellow-green including red, orange-red, orange, orange-yellow, and yellow. The warm hues are also known as highlighting tones because they are the colors that reflect rather than absorb more light.

To warm a formulation, add the next warmest color on the circle. To create maximum warmth, add pure red. Red is the "hottest" color on the circle.

Cool hues are those from red-violet to yellow-green going in the opposite direction. The cool hues include violet, blue-violet, blue, blue-green, and green. The cool hues are also known as ash or drab tones. The technical term "drab," is not used in client consultation. It carries a negative connotation that does not sell color.

To cool a formulation, add the next cooler color on the wheel. To create maximum drabbing effect, add pure blue. Blue is the "coldest" color on the wheel.

Complementary Colors

The term "complementary" comes from the word "complement," which means to make complete or to mutually make up what is lacking. When using the additive method of color mixing, the term "complementary color" indicates any two colors of the spectrum that combine to form white or whitish light. In other words, the two colors mutually make up the ingredients necessary to make white light. *(See Color Plate 7.)*

When using the subtractive method of color mixing, the color directly across the Chromatic Circle mutually makes up the ingredients missing to create a neutral hue. *(See Color Plate 8.)* Complementary colors are those positioned on the Chromatic Circle directly across from each other. Green is opposite red, orange is opposite blue, violet is opposite yellow. When using pigments, many professionals prefer to call these colors neutralizing colors.

Neutralizing Effect of Complementary Colors

According to the Laws of Color, these hues that are positioned directly across from each other on the Chromatic Circle, when mixed in equal proportions, will neutralize each other. *(See Color Plate 9.)* Green neutralizes red. Orange neutralizes blue. Violet neutralizes yellow.

Neutralization creates a color that is neutral in tone rather than warm or cool. Pigments of a low level mixed in this manner will create black. Pure true pigments in a higher (lighter) level will create shades of gray. Neither the resulting gray or black will have predominant tones that are either warm or cool. *(See Color Plate 10.)*

The colors manufactured for colorists to work with are not true, pure pigments. Hair colors generally are "balanced" colors to prevent the accidental occurrence of purple or turquoise hair. A balanced color contains a predominant color by which the product is located on the Chromatic Circle. However, it will also contain small amounts of undertones of the remaining primary hues to create a balance. Because of this, the netural tones achieved when mixing hair color range from black to shades of brown to light beige depending upon the level of color used. *(See Color Plate 11.)*

Dab a small amount of the appropriate color next to its name on the *Neutralization with Complementary Colors* chart. Mix the hues listed below on a piece of waxed paper to create a neutralizing effect and then place a dab of the neutralized hue after the = sign.

NEUTRALIZATION WITH COMPLEMENTARY COLORS

Green	+	Red	=	
Blue-green	+	Orange-red	=	
Blue	+	Orange	=	
Blue-violet	+	Gold	=	
Violet	+	Yellow	=	
Red-violet	+	Yellow-green	=	
Red	+	Green	=	
Orange-red	+	Blue-green	=	
Orange	+	Blue	=	
Gold	+	Blue-violet	=	
Yellow	+	Violet	=	
Yellow-green	+	Red-violet	=	

Level Adjustment

The level of any hue can be adjusted by the addition of white or black. To experience this concept place small dabs of the three primary colors on a piece of waxed paper.

Paint the center circle of each primary grouping with the primary hue indicated. On the waxed paper, add a tiny amount of black to a dab of pure red and a larger amount of white to a different dab of pure red. Paint the adjusted level on the circles as labeled.

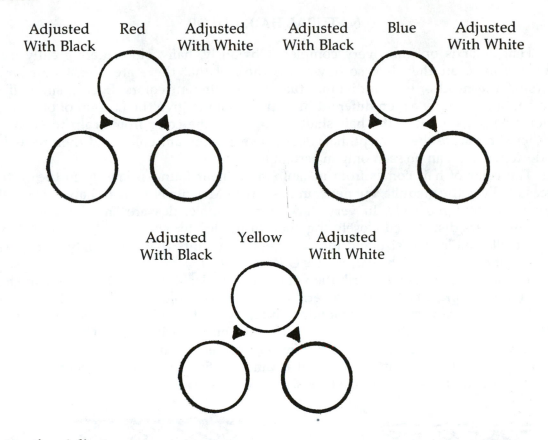

Saturation Adjustment

Saturation is adjusted by the addition of more of the same color. To experience this concept, paint the entire square *lightly* with the primary indicated. Let dry. Apply a second application over ¾ of the square. Let dry. Apply a third application over ½ of the square. Let dry. Apply a fourth application over ¼ of the square. Let dry. Observe the differences in the intensity or saturation of the hue.

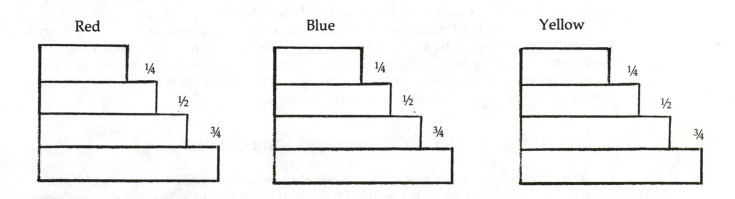

A working knowledge of The Artist's Concept of the Laws of Color will enable the professional colorist to create any desired hue, regardless of level or saturation. This ability opens the doors to a whole new world of color. *(See Color Plate 12.)*

NATURAL HAIR COLOR

Hair color is optically very complex. Obviously, hair color differs greatly from one person to another. Not so obvious is the fact that there are a vast number of hairs on the head of each individual that are of different colors. Even a single fiber can contain as many as ten different hues that blend to give the illusion of one single color. Then again, often the hair shaft is not the same color from scalp to ends. To further complicate the concept, hair fibers have a dominant color, and then recessive undertones that can be seen only in certain lights.

The color of hair comes from melanin, a pigment found primarily in the cortex, occasionally in the medulla, but never in the cuticle. Melanin is an oval shaped, blackish-brown pigment molecule. In very dark hair the molecules are large and found in great numbers distributed closely together. In the lighter shades of hair the melanin is of smaller molecular size and found in lesser amounts that are widely distributed througout the length of the cortex. *(See Color Plates 13-19.)*

The size, amount, and distribution of melanin molecules throughout the hair shaft are the predominant factors that determine natural hair color by reflecting light waves that the brain interprets as hues blonde to black, warm to cool. However, the melanin's position deep within the hair strand also contributes to its color. The light waves of the visible spectrum of color are diffused by the translucent cuticle. The greater the layers of cuticle, the more the light is diffused, first one way and then the other as it bounces off the many cuticle layers.

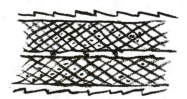

Intermittent medulla of blonde hair.

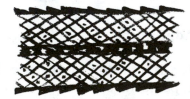

Solid medulla of black or dark brown hair.

The medulla affects the hair color by the amount of light either reflected or absorbed by its presence. The more color absorbed, the darker the strand will appear. The more medulla, the more light absorbed. The fact that blonde hair generally has little or no medulla contributes to the fact that it is blonde. The light is reflected through the cuticle with little or no absorption by the medulla. The inability of current hair coloring technology to recreate this phenomenon is the reason that artificially colored hair never looks quite the same as the natural color.

ANALYZING NATURAL HAIR COLOR

The natural hair color provides the base upon which artificial color will react; therefore, correct analysis of the natural hair color is crucial to achieving the desired results. Clean, dry hair is necessary because hair that is either dirty or damp will appear darker and can influence the colorist's decisions. Good lighting is also crucial to correct selection, as fluorescent lighting will cool the appearance of a color while incandescent lighting will make it appear warmer than it really is. Natural lighting gives the most accurate reading of color. The next concept that must be mastered for successful color analysis is "The Level System."

The Level System

The Level System is a method of measuring and comparing a color in relation to its lightness and darkness. This method is used to identify the depth of both natural and artificial color. The Level System is crucial to formulating, matching, and correcting colors.

The lighter the color, the higher it is ranked in the system. For example, lightest blonde is ranked as level 10. The darker the color, the lower it is ranked. Black is ranked as level 1. The intermediate colors are ranked in between 1 and 10 according to their depth. *(See Color Plate 20.)*

THE LEVEL SYSTEM

Level 10—Lightest blonde
Level 9—Very light blonde
Level 8—Light blonde
Level 7—Medium blonde
Level 6—Dark blonde
Level 5—Lightest brown
Level 4—Light brown
Level 3—Medium brown
Level 2—Dark brown
Level 1—Black

While level is only one characteristic, it is the most difficult to learn to identify and the most important to the outcome of the color process. The level system can be learned by working with any manufacturer's level identification swatches or natural hair swatches. Then use the following simple steps as a guide to determine the level of the natural color.

Establishing the Level of Natural Color

1. Determine the color group by identifying whether the natural color falls in the blonde or brown grouping on the Level System.
2. Select the three colors that are similar to the color of the hair swatch matching the natural hair color.
3. Spread the swatches out.
4. Eliminate the most obvious.
5. Squint. Squinting tends to block out tone and saturation, thus making it easier to identify the level.
6. Make your final selection.

Identifying Tonality of Natural Color

Identifying the tone is a simpler process than that of the level. Tone falls into two categories: *cool* and *warm*.

The cool colors are also known as "drab" or "ash." To identify a cool color, look for an absence of warmth. The cool colors reflect a blue, violet, or green undertone. They will appear less shiny than warm colors, but most important to color identification, cool colors absorb more light rays and therefore appear darker to the eye than warm colors.

The warm colors are also known as "highlighters" or "oxidized colors." To identify a warm color, look for the presence of yellow, gold, orange, red or any combination thereof. Because of the great amount of light they reflect, the warm colors tend to look lighter and shinier than the cool colors.

Predictable Tonalities

Certain tonalities are more common in particular levels of color. The dark, light absorbing colors may not reflect enough light for the eye to read the tone. However, it is still there and may be referred to as an "undertone."

Listed below is a guide that the colorist may use as a training tool in learning to distinguish and identify tone.

NATURAL LEVEL	TONE
10 Lightest blonde	Yellow
9 Very light blonde	Yellow
8 Light blonde	Yellow-gold
7 Medium blonde	Gold, orange, or green
6 Dark blonde	Gold, orange, or green
5 Lightest brown	Gold, orange-red, or green
4 Light brown	Gold, orange, red, or green
3 Medium brown	Orange, red, or green
2 Dark brown	Red or violet
1 Black	Blue or violet

Condition and Texture of Hair

An excessively oily condition of the scalp and hair will slightly impede the processing of hair color. Hair that is not coated with sebum will process slightly faster. This can result in unpredictable results. A normal amount of oiliness will be dissolved by the surfactants and solvents within the product. However, if the hair is extremely coated with sebum, pre-shampooing is recommended.

The strength of the hair is governed by the structure of the cortical layer of the shaft. Many clients have hair that is not strong enough to receive a hair coloring service due to excessive chemical treatments and styling techniques. When the natural bonds and pigments within the cortex are excessively damaged, a penetrating color will not be able to form and attach properly within the cortex. Thus the color service will produce undesired and unexpected results such as off-tones or incorrect level development.

The cortical layer is also responsible for elasticity. Color has a drying quality and tends to slightly reduce elasticity. Under normal conditions, this causes no problem but if the elastic properties of the hair are already poor, a color may cause the hair to reach the point that when stretched, it will not return to its original length, or it may even snap and break.

The cuticle protects the cortex from damage. The cuticle is normally quite strong and resistant to chemical and physical damage. However, an abused cuticle indicates over porosity that will effect hair color results. A raised or partially removed cuticle allows permanent and semipermanent colors to penetrate faster than intended by the manufacturer. Because of this, the color will become excessively dark. Rapid fading also occurs because the cuticle cannot close back down tightly to hold in the artificial color pigment.

Damaged or missing cuticle also allows coating colors to penetrate when they are not intended to. This creates staining, grabbing, and off-tones on this over-porous hair.

If a great deal of cuticle has been removed at the end of the hair shaft, the cuticle becomes exposed and frayed, a condition commonly known as a "split end." This damaged condition at the ends will "grab" color and become stained and darker than the rest of the shaft.

The texture of the hair must also be considered when planning the steps for successful color. Normally coarse hair is strong hair. It can undergo almost any coloring service without excessive damage as long as the correct chemicals and procedures are used.

Fine hair, on the other hand, is fragile hair and must be handled with care. While coloring does make the hair coarser and thereby creates more body and manageability, it can be naturally too delicate for drastic level changes such as taking a level 2 or 3 to a level 10.

Normal hair is the "middle-of-the-road" type. It is generally stronger than fine and weaker than coarse hair. Most hair coloring treatments performed under professional supervision can be successful on normal hair.

COLOR SYSTEMS

A color system refers to the classification of color and the system it uses to achieve the manufacturer's intended purpose. For example, a temporary color system is used for the purpose of deposition only.

After the natural level and tone are established, the next step to successful color is to compare them to the color the client desires as established in the client consultation. The colorist must at this time determine the type of hair color system to be used. A study of the various color systems (bleaches, tints, rinses) is necessary to provide the background knowledge to make this decision. However, the following chart gives a brief overview.

CLASSIFICATION	ACTION
Temporary	Deposition only
Semipermanent	Deposition only
Permanent tint:	
10 or less volume	Deposition only
20 volume peroxide	Normal lift (2 levels) and deposition
30 volume peroxide	Lifts 3 levels—some deposition
40 volume peroxide	Lifts 4 levels—little deposition
Oil bleach	Lifts 2-3 levels
Cream bleach	Lifts through all levels of color
Powder bleach	Lifts through all levels of color

"Color balance" is a term that refers to the balance of pigments within the color of a particular system that creates the finished hue on the head. Few hair colorings are made of one primary pigment. Most are a balance of the three primaries. One color is generally predominant with smaller proportions of the other two to give a balance of hue that simulates natural hair color.

"Pigment weight" refers to the molecular weight of the artificial pigment that is being deposited on or in the hair shaft. Basically, the more temporary the color, the larger the molecular size of the pigment. Bleaches generally have no pigment to be deposited.

The chemical composition varies greatly from one color system to the other. The colorist must have a working knowledge of this composition and its safety factors to provide professional services. These factors are discussed in depth in the chapter covering each individual color system.

DYES AND PIGMENTS

Manufacturers of hair colorings use a wide variety of dyes and pigments to formulate their products. These organic and inorganic colorants are mixed and combined to create an uncountable number of chemical formulas for use in all classifications of color. For the most part, use of dyes and pigments for hair coloring has been adapted from other industry uses, such as to color fur, fabric, food, rubber, and plastic.

A dye is a colorant that dissolves or disperses in water or a solvent. It is added to a solution and then applied to a medium (fur, fabric, hair) to which it gives color.

Logwood is the only natural dye that is still in production on a large scale, but its use in hair color is rare. Synthetic dyes are the types of dyes most commonly used in hair coloring products. The earliest synthetic dyes were obtained from aniline taken from coal tar through a complicated two-step process of separation and preparation. Many synthetic dyes currently in use are obtained from petroleum sources through a process that incorporates boiling and treatment with other chemicals. The change is largely due to the replacement of coal gas by natural gas.

The primary types of dyes used in the beauty industry are acid dyes, basic dyes, direct dyes, disperse dyes, developed dyes, pre-metallized dyes, reactive dyes, and vat dyes. Each type of dye is defined below and followed by examples used in the hair color industry.

Acid Dyes—Acid dyes are dissolved in acid solutions. They have a molecular structure that is similar to keratin. Some colors achieved with acid dyes remain stable and fast; others do not. Those providing the best water and light fastness are compounds including metals. In addition to their use in hair color products, acid dyes provide an inexpensive dye for varnishes and plastics as well as creating saturated hues for nylon, silk, and wool.

- Acid black 131
- Acid blue 62
- Acid brown 48
- Acid green 25 (D&C green no. 25)
- Acid violet 43 (D&C violet no. 2)
- Pigment red 4 (D&C red no. 36)
- Pigment red 53 (D&C red no. 8)
- Pigment red 53:1 (D&C red no. 9)
- Pigment red 63:1 (D&C red no. 34)
- Pigment red 64:1 (D&C red no. 31)
- Pigment red 112
- Pigment yellow 1, 3, 12, 13, 73
- Pigment violet 19

Basic Dyes—Basic dyes also have a molecular structure similar to that of keratin. They are not extremely colorfast but exhibit improved staying power when formulated in conjunction with tannic acid. Basic dyes are chemically known as cationic dyes. These dyes are made from soluble salts, minerals, and organic salts. They produce bright colors for use in hair color, acrylic, wool, and other fibers. They exhibit all the toxicity and allergy characteristics of aniline.

- Acid blue 9 (FD&C blue no. 1)
- Acid blue 9 ammonium salt (D&C no. 4)
- Acid red 51 (FD&C red no. 3)
- Acid red 52
- Acid red 87 (D&C red no. 22)
- Acid red 92 (D&C red no. 28)
- Acid red 95 (D&C orange no. 11)
- FD&C blue no. 1
- FD&C green nos. 1, 2, 3

Direct Dyes—Direct dyes color without the help of a mordant, although salt is added to achieve deep levels of hue. Direct dyes are often combined with aniline in hair dyes to improve their fastness. Direct dyes are a common colorant of cotton and rayon. The azo, monoazo, disazo, and trisazo dyes fall in this category.

- Acid black 107 (lanamed black BL)
- Acid orange 7 (D&C orange no. 4)
- Acid orange 24 (D&C brown no. 1)
- Acid red 33 (D&C red no. 33)
- Acid red 35 (a positive animal carcinogen)
- FD&C red no. 40 (allura red AC.)
- Direct brown 1 (benzochrome, brown G, benzamine brown)
- Direct red 81 (benzo fast)

Disperse Dyes—Disperse dyes dissolve only slightly in water. For the most part they just spread out or disperse. Dyeing at high temperatures helps dissolve the insoluble dye particles into fabrics, resins, and waxes. In hair coloring, a preheated dryer assists with the color development. Sulfated oils are also added in hair color formulas to help disperse the dye.

- Disperse black 9
- Disperse blue 1
- Disperse yellow 1, 3

Developed Dyes—Developed dyes involve a reaction of two colorless chemicals to produce a deeply colored dye in the medium. The reaction in oxidation tints between the intermediate and the coupler creates a developed dye. (See Oxidation Tints.) This chemical reaction produces a deeply colored hair fiber. It also increases the brightness and colorfastness in acrylic, cotton, nylon, and rayon.

- Acid yellow 73 (D&C yellow no. 7)
- Ext. D&C yellow no. 7
- Ext. D&C yellow no. 7 (aluminum lake)
- FD&C blue no. 1 (brilliant blue)
- FD&C blue no. 2
- FD&C red no. 3 (erythrosine)

Pre-Metallized Dyes—Pre-metallized dyes contain metals such as lead, chromium, and copper to improve color fastness. Pre-metallized dyes have the ability to lower the quality of the natural keratin content of the hair or any protein content of the formula. They create a one stage coloring that offers little control of color result. In addition to their use in hair color, pre-metallized dyes are widely used on acrylic, nylon, and wool. Metals such as the ones listed below are added to other classifications of dyes and pigments to create pre-metallized dyes.

- Copper sulfate
- Iron oxides
- Lead acetate
- Zinc acetate
- Zinc carbonate
- Zinc oxide
- Zinc sulfide
- Zirconium

Reactive Dyes—Reactive dyes form a strong chemical bond within the hair fiber. They are effective in cold alkaline conditions. They are also used to create bright colors in cotton, nylon, and rayon.

- HC blue nos. 1, 2, 3, 4
- HC brown no.1
- HC orange no. 1
- HC red nos. 1, 3, 6
- HC yellow nos. 2, 3, 4, 5

Vat Dyes—Vat dye refers to a liquid containing a dye that does not color the materials dipped into it until they are exposed to air. Vat dyes, among the most colorfast of all dyes, are popular for use on cotton and rayon. These organic compounds are considered to be low in toxicity.

- Chamomile
- Acid yellow 23 (D&C yellow no. 5)
- FD&C yellow no. 5 (tartrazine)
- Indigo
- Tyrolean purple
- Vat red 1 (D&C red no. 30 aluminum lake)
- Violet extract
- Walnut extract

Pigments—Pigments are small, solid particles that do not dissolve in the prepared hair coloring solution. They simply spread out. Pigments differ from dyes in that their chemical structure bears no similarity or relationship to keratin. Because of this, they do not readily affix to the hair. To correct this problem, an adhesive is generally included in a formula that uses pigments.

Inorganic pigments
- Acid yellow 1 (D&C yellow no. 7)
- Ultramarine blue
- Ultramarine green
- Ultramarine pink
- Ultramarine violet

Organic Pigments
- Pigment yellow 1
- FD&C yelow no. 5 aluminum lake
- FD&C yellow no. 6 aluminum lake

THE NEED TO UNDERSTAND CHEMICAL COMPOSITION

Over 2,000 different companies manufacture or distribute beauty products in the United States alone. Even the Federal Government does not know how many companies exist or how many products they produce, much less what ingredients are used and if they are safe.

The advertising claims on hair coloring packages, or any other industry product for that matter, should be read with caution. General claims such as "conditioning action" or "shampoo in color" are sometimes misleading.

Relying on the advice of the salesperson should not be the only method of learning about a hair color. Scientifically researched and well practiced sales pitches often have little to do with the reality of using the product on a client. Therefore, it becomes necessary for the colorist to become knowledgeable as to the chemical composition of the products they use.

HOW TO READ THE INGREDIENTS LIST

Ingredients are listed in descending order. The first ingredient will make up the largest proportion of the product, and the last ingredient will make up the smallest. This gives quite a bit of information to help the colorist provide professional services.

However, this information is incomplete because many professional products are not required to list ingredients and the FDA accepts "trade secrets" that are not required to be divulged. The manufacturer does not even have to list the fact that there are undisclosed chemicals in the product. Nor is it required to list the amount of each ingredient in the formula. The facts and figures that the manufacturer is *not* required to divulge can alter the results the colorist might expect after reading the ingredients listed on the product. For example, consider the two semipermanent color formulas below:

FORMULA I	*FORMULA II*
Water	Water
Butoxyethanol	Butoxyethanol
Cocamide dea	Cocamide dea
Hydroxylethylcellulose	Hydroxylethylcellulose
Undisclosed ingredients	Undisclosed ingredients

The formulas appear to be identical. However, in many ways, they may differ greatly. The ingredients list may be composed of the identical chemicals in the same descending order, but the amount of each can vary from one formula to the other. Reconsider this same formula with the percentages added.

FORMULA I	*FORMULA II*
60% Water	90% Water
20% Butoxyethanol	4% Butoxyethanol
12% Cocamide dea	3% Cocamide dea
5% Hydroxylethylcellulose	2% Hydroxylethylcellulose
3% Undisclosed ingredients	1% Undisclosed ingredients

It now becomes easy to see that the formulas are not nearly as identical as the original listing implied. Other formulation variables that are not shared with the professional colorist may also affect the performance of a product. Technical procedures such as blending, quality, purity, molecular size, mixing time, and cooling time may make one product favorable over another.

Because these factors are not freely shared by the manufacturers, performing a test strand to become familiar with new products is crucial to the education of the colorist. You may also write the manufacturer to request the "Materials Safety Data Sheet" for individual products. Through testing of products on hair swatches and studying available chemical information, the colorist can achieve a truly professional level of providing safe and reliable services to the public.

HOW TO DO A COLORING EXPERIMENT

You can read this book, and every other hair coloring book for that matter, until the pages fall out and still not *know* how to color hair. Learning is a kinetic activity that requires more than just reading and thinking. A thorough knowledge of the theory and chemistry of color is crucial as most mistakes occur because the colorist did not think the situation through. However, you will not really be an expert until you can utilize color successfully in any manner of your choosing.

Hair Swatches

The most efficient and safe way to learn hair coloring is on hair swatches. All major manufacturers recommend the use of hair swatches to become familiar with their product. Swatches provide the medium for a great variety of experiments on different types and shades of hair. With a handful of hair, it is possible to test an entire line of colors and compare the results without risking loss of clients. The completed hair swatches can then become sales tools. Clients feel more comfortable selecting a color they can see and touch on real hair than they do selecting one from pictures in a book.

The step-by-step procedures described in this book must be followed to obtain results on the swatches that will be comparable to live model applications. It is extremely frustrating to do these experiments and have them fail or not be comparable to industry standards because the swatches were not properly prepared.

Supplies Needed

- Quick drying glue or clear nail polish
- Timer
- Waterproof ink pen
- Hair dryer
- Waxed paper or potato wrap
- Experiment sheet
- Hair (preferably virgin)
- Color products
- Masking tape

Type of Hair to Use

Mannequin, wig, and hairpiece strands, as well as most commercially prepared hair swatches, are already tinted or bleached. For a few experiments, this is acceptable, but for the majority of the learning experiences in this book, virgin hair is required.

Virgin hair in this case means hair that has not been treated with any other permanent hair coloring treatment. Temporary rinses, permanent waves, and relaxers are prior chemical treatments that will not interfere with the experiment results as long as the hair is in good condition.

The strands of hair in each swatch should be at least 2 inches in length and thick enough to make a swatch as big around as a pencil. These are minimums. The swatches can always be longer and thicker. The more substantial the swatch, the easier it is to accurately access and compare color results.

Where to Find Hair

Your best source of hair is the neighborhood salons and schools. If you wait for haircuts on your friends and family members to provide you with enough swatches, you will be ready to retire before you have enough hair to learn the things you need to know to be a successful colorist. Other students and stylists generally are willing to help you acquire hair—if you remind them regularly.

Gray and salt-and-pepper hair are often the most difficult shades to collect. A trip to the local convalescent hospital to offer complimentary hair cuts is a good way to acquire a variety of shades of mature hair.

Storing the Hair

Dry the hair thoroughly to keep it from mildewing. Store it in plastic bags to keep it clean. Lay the hair out straight in the bag with the freshly cut ends together. If the hair is allowed to twist and become mixed, the cuticles will rub and lock, causing the hair to tangle. However, the worst tangling will occur when the hair becomes wet.

Be sure that you can tell which end of the hair is freshly cut before you are ready to prepare the swatches for experimentation. Wigs, hairpieces, and mannequins that have the hair attached at the free ends instead of the cut ends are known as "root tied." If you encounter such a hairpiece, you will recognize it immediately. When wet it will mat up like a wet dog and you will either spend hours combing it out, strand by strand, or you will trash the whole thing. Conditioner and cream rinses have little or no effect on hair that is root tied.

Hair swatches attached at the free ends will react just like a hairpiece that is root tied. They will mat so badly that by the time you get them combed out, there is not enough hair left to see your color results! So be sure to put all the freshly cut ends together.

Making the Swatches

Coat the scalp end of the hair swatch with quick drying glue or clear nail polish and let it harden. The swatches are now ready to color.

Labeling the Swatches

Color experiments lose a great deal of their value if, upon completion, the colorist cannot determine which color went on which strand, how long it was left on, or what the formula was. To each swatch, attach a piece of masking tape over the glued end. With a waterproof marking pen write enough information on the masking tape to identify the swatch when it is time to mount it on the experiment sheet. For example, one swatch might be labeled: *Bleach Experiment—Cream*, while the second swatch would be labeled: *Bleach Experiment—Powder*.

Formulation

While using this text, the formulations are explained in detail or directions are given to follow the manufacturers' recommended directions. Upon completion of this text, you will want to continue on your own to experiment, to learn and grow in the field of color. Accurately measure and record all experiments so that they can be duplicated (or possibly never duplicated again, as in the case of some color discoveries).

Safety

Always wear gloves when working with hair coloring products. The cosmetologist is very susceptible to allergies and adverse reactions from working with these chemicals because of their repeated use.

Follow manufacturers' recommended directions for each individual product.

Preparation

For protection of the work area, cover it with several layers of waxed paper. Mix products in nonmetallic receptacles.

Product Application

Lay the strands out on either waxed paper or potato wrap. Contrary to popular belief, aluminum foil is not acceptable. The metallic content of aluminum foil causes hydrogen peroxide to liberate its gases at a more rapid rate than is normal, thus creating inaccurate and unpredictable color results.

The coloring product must be applied to both sides of the hair swatch and worked into the strand for even processing. Particular care is needed to achieve even color application in the area where the glue has bunched the hair strand together. If the product is not applied to the entire strand, interior and exterior, the finished product will have leopard spots. The thicker the product, the more difficult it is to thoroughly saturate the inner strands of hair. The thinner products will ooze somewhat during processing. Those with the thicker consistency tend to stay where they are put; therefore, products such as bleach need extra care in the application.

Do not wrap the swatch tightly in the waxed paper or potato wrap *unless* the application on the client will involve covering the product such as is done in weaving and frosting. Enclosing the saturated swatch increases the heat and causes the color to process quicker than it would if left open. This will distort the accuracy of your experiments.

Do not put the swatches under a dryer unless that is the standard method of using the product on a client. If the coloring product dries out, the processing stops. If it remains moist, this type of extreme heat accelerates the color to unpredictable results. Place the swatches out of the draft from a door, window, heating, or air-conditioning vent and keep it moderately warm to simulate the body heat. A manicuring light will simulate body heat if it is not placed too close to the hair.

Timing

The timing will vary from experiment to experiment. Therefore, it is crucial that each experiment is accurately timed and recorded if the results are ever to be duplicated.

When doing color experimentations on hair swatches, it is necessary to compensate for the time that would be spent applying the product to the entire head. For this reason, in these experiments, add 10 minutes to the manufacturers' recommended timing. For example, if the manufacturer states that the product processes in 25 minutes, leave the color on the swatch for 35 minutes. This compensates for the 10 minutes that a professional generally takes to apply an entire head application.

Product Removal

It is important to treat a swatch just as if it were an entire head of hair coloring. This means to shampoo *twice* to remove all traces of color, rinse thoroughly, apply a pH balancer, and then dry the swatch before mounting it in your book. If the process is not completely stopped, a slight oxidation process can continue for as long as 72 hours and the next time you look at your swatches, the color may have altered!

Also, if the swatches are put in the book wet, they mildew, they get bent and mangled looking, the color rubs off on the pages, the pages stick together, and the ink runs through so you cannot read the next page. Trust me. It can become a big mess.

Mounting the Swatches

Each experiment has a special page for mounting and labeling. Cut on the dotted lines and slide the swatch through. Tape it on the back so that the tape does not show. Fill in all the blanks on product information and make any additional comments that will help you with future use of the color.

Examine the colors like a doctor does a new patient. Compare them in sunlight, fluorescent, and incandescent light. Record your impressions of how the colors change in the different types of light waves. Analyze the color change of the swatch. Is it darker, lighter, warmer, cooler, or a combination of more than one characteristic? Record the condition and texture changes. The more experienced you become with color, the more you will be able to use this information to create future formulations.

2
Hair Coloring Applications

Hair coloring applications all fall into two main classifications: *single-process coloring* and *double-process coloring.*

Single-process coloring achieves the desired result with a single application. The application itself may incorporate several steps, but one application creates the desired color. Single-process coloring is also known as single-application coloring, one-step coloring, one-step tinting, and single-application tinting.

Examples of single-process coloring are:

- Virgin tint applications
- Tint retouch applications
- Semipermanent rinse applications
- Temporary color applications

Double-process coloring requires two separate and distinct applications to achieve the desired color. Double-process coloring is also known as double-application coloring, two-step coloring, two-step tinting, and double-application tinting.

Examples of double-process coloring are:

- Bleach and toner applications
- Presoftening and tinting applications
- Filler and tint applications

THREE CLASSIFICATIONS OF HAIR COLOR

Hair color is divided into three classifications: *temporary, semipermanent,* and *permanent.* These classifications indicate color fastness or ability to remain on the hair. These characteristics are determined by chemical composition and molecular weight of the pigments and dyes within the products found in each classification.

Temporary colors utilize pigment and dye molecules of the greatest molecular weight, making these molecules the largest used in the three classifications of hair color. The large size of this color molecule prevents penetration of the cuticle layer of the hair shaft and allows only a coating action on the outside of the strand.

The chemical composition of a temporary color is acid in reaction and makes only a physical change rather than a chemical change in the shaft. This creates a color that is designed to be removed completely with the next shampooing.

Semipermanent pigment and dye molecules are of a lesser molecular weight than those of temporary colors. These smaller molecules have the physical capability to penetrate the hair shaft somewhat. The chemical composition of semipermanent colors is mildly alkaline in reaction, thus causing the cortex to swell and the cuticle to raise to allow some penetration. This mild alkaline solution, combined with a mild oxidizer, creates a classification of color that becomes "self-penetrating."

The semipermanent colors make a mild chemical change as well as a physical change. These changes create a color designed to be removed gradually through shampooing, leaving behind a slight diffusion of color that often goes unnoticed by the human eye.

THREE CLASSIFICATIONS OF COLOR

	Temporary	Semipermanent	Permanent
Molecular weight of dye molecule	Large	Medium	Small
pH	Acid	Slightly alkaline	Alkaline
Reaction or change	Physical	Chemical & physical	Chemical & physical
Color fastness	Removed with shampooing	Fades gradually	Permanent
Color changes	Deposits	Deposits	Lightens & deposits

The pigment and dye molecules of the permanent oxidation coloring have the lowest molecular weight, making them the smallest used in the three classifications of hair color. These molecules are small enough to enter through the cuticle and penetrate deep into the cortex, creating a color as permanent as current technology allows.

Permanent tints are alkaline in reaction. This creates a chemical process that causes the cortex to swell, thus raising and separating the cuticle so that the small pigment and dye molecules can enter the shaft. After the addition of a full strength oxidizer, the product is able to diffuse melanin as the artificial color molecules swell and become a part of the structure of the cortex. As the color is shampooed and dried, it begins to return to its normal pH. This causes the cortex to shrink and the cuticle to close. The color molecules become trapped beneath the cuticle. Even though the color fades eventually, the cortex undergoes permanent chemical and structural changes.

TEMPORARY HAIR COLOR

The classification of temporary hair coloring encompasses all methods in which the pigment and dye molecules are intended to be completely removed from the outside of the hair shaft with one shampoo. In addition to the use of a large pigment molecule, the acidic chemical formulation of these colors does not allow for penetration of the hair shaft. These two factors allow only color deposition. No temporary color will lighten natural or artificial color. A wide variety of products are available within this classification: color rinses (instant and concentrated), color shampoos, color sprays, color gels, mousses, and creams, color crayons, mascara, and color powders.

TEMPORARY COLOR RINSES

History

Prior to the manufacture of shampoos made of synthetic detergents, soap was used to cleanse the hair. Soap leaves a curd on the outside of the hair shaft that tends to dull the hair even after extensive rinsing with clear water. To remove this curd it became common practice to rinse the hair with vinegar or lemon juice. This acid rinse neutralized the alkali and restored the natural highlights of the hair.

This same principle was used to formulate temporary colorants with a solution of citric or tartaric acid. The most well-known of these early rinses, the *Nestle Rinse*, was developed by LeMur in the 1920's from fabric dye. These rinses consisted of a mixture of powdered acid and dyestuff packaged in a plastic capsule. The powder was mixed with hot water and poured repeatedly over freshly shampooed hair. It removed soap curd as it toned the hair.

Contemporary Uses

Now that soap has been replaced by synthetic detergents, temporary rinses are used mainly for their ability to affect the color of the hair rather than to remove soap curd. A wide range of uses, gentleness on the hair, economical cost, and ease of application make temporary color rinses sought for both professional and home use.

Temporary rinses are also known as water rinses within the industry. The term water rinse refers to the chemical composition of a temporary rinse, which is a formula of either a simple aqueous or aqueous-alcoholic solution combined with a variety of dyestuffs.

Color Selection

Temporary rinses are available in natural shades, toning hues, as well as the bright, vibrant colors of the artist's palette. Because they have no lasting effect, temporary rinses offer clients the advantage of giving colors a "trial run." Even though these rinses do not give the depth or saturation of color available with semipermanent or permanent tints, they do allow clients to see themselves in a comparable shade of hair color. In this manner, temporary rinses serve as an effective sales tool to introduce clients to the world of hair color.

The natural looking shades of temporary rinses are often used to intensify the present tinted or natural hair color that has faded or become streaked. These rinses can be used as a refresher in between regular touch-ups, or they can provide welcome relief from the boredom of wearing exactly the same hair color week after week.

Warm, cool, and neutral hues are available in a variety of levels and saturations and the temporary colors can be mixed together to create customized color as well. This versatility makes it easy to select a color to suit any client's needs.

Gray hair lends itself well to the use of temporary color rinses. They will not give complete coverage of gray, but rinses do tone and blend the lighter strands to make them less noticeable or to camouflage yellow off-tones.

A variety of pale colors, similar to the shades of permanent toners, are available in the form of temporary rinses. They are used to cool excessive yellow and warm undesirable ash tones in pre-lightened hair.

Temporary rinses are particularly useful to change the tone of the bleached strands of frosted or weaved hair. The application of a hydrogen peroxide toner on the unbleached strands would lighten and possibly create undesirable brass on the unbleached strands. This same principle is applicable to an entire head of bleached and toned hair that now has a regrowth. The application of a peroxide toner to refresh the color would process the regrowth to the orange stage, thus creating a need for corrective color.

The pastel shades of this acid color rinse also assist in preventing alkali degradation after bleaching. This characteristic lends credibility to claims that temporary rinses can be considered to have conditioning qualities.

In addition to the wide selection of natural and toning shades, a smaller group of high fashion colors are available in temporary rinses. This classification of hair color enables even the most timid to experiment with turquoise or violet streaks without risk. Temporary rinses have stimulated a never ending market for those who dare to wear the avant-garde on a regular basis as well as those who just want an occasional change of hue.

In comparison with other coloring services and products, temporary color rinses are economical. The cost of the bulk product is reasonable and the small amount of time and skill necessary for application keeps it within the reach of most clients. The porosity of the hair shaft must be considered when selecting a temporary rinse. Color selection can be a problem when there are differences in the porosity from the root to the ends of the hair shaft. The areas that are nonporous will hold little color, the areas that are over-porous will hold a great deal of color, and the areas of average porosity will hold a normal amount of color. This uneven coverage can result in a variety of streaky or blotchy looks.

A second problem can occur due to over-porosity. The raised cuticle can "grab" the base color of the rinse rather than achieving the finished hue intended by the manufacturer. Also, hair that is so porous as to have lost some of its own melanin does not offer the appropriate base colors to blend with the hue of the temporary pigment. This results in the reflection of wavelengths that the eye interprets differently than the intended hue. While purple, gray, and green are the three most common off-tones that occur, any base shade can appear when these temporary rinses are used on over-porous hair.

More than one shampoo is generally needed to remove the temporary rinse molecules that grab into the raised or removed cuticle. If the tones will not shampoo out, then use the Chromatic Circle to neutralize them.

The rinse can also build up as it is trapped by the roughened cuticle if the shampoo used is not strong enough to open the cuticle layers and remove the color. When a rinse or its base color will not loosen with normal shampoo, use a more alkaline shampoo to strip off the build-up. However, if either the stain or build-up is particularly resistant, it may be necessary to use an oil-based color remover, as described in *Oil Base Color Removers on page 159*.

All temporary rinses tend to rub off onto combs, brushes, pillowcases, and sometimes the collar of the wearer. The darker the shade, the more noticeable the rub-off.

Use of Gloves

Temporary color rinses will stain the colorist's hands unless the hue is of a very low level and saturation. The pigment molecules are designed to attach to hard keratin. Skin and hair are composed of similar types of keratin, the skin being soft keratin and the hair being hard. Soft keratin is even more reactive than the hard, allowing rinses to stain the scalp as well as the skin.

Another faactor that contributes to the staining of hands is the fact that the cosmetologist's skin is generally over-porous due to continued exposure to water, detergents, and other chemicals. The large pigment molecule of this product can easily slip under the dry, damaged stratum corneum layer of the epidermis. Therefore, it is advisable to wear gloves when applying this color product even though it has a low incidence of allergy and toxicity.

Two Types of Temporary Rinses

Two types of temporary color rinses are currently available: *instant* and *concentrated*. The instant color rinses are popular for their ease of use. They are applied as packaged in the bottle and remain in the hair like a styling gel. Instant rinses are available in a wide variety of colors that are economical to purchase.

Concentrated rinses are mixed with hot water before application and must be rinsed from the hair after remaining for a 5 to 10 minute processing time. The concentrated rinses have a limited range of color selection. While traces of the dark shades of both types of rinses can be seen on combs, brushes, pillowcases, and collars, the concentrated seem to show less rub-off because the excess is rinsed off before the hair is styled.

Chemical Composition

Water is the first on the ingredient list of the instant rinses. This means that there is more water in this formulation than any other one ingredient in the product. If the water is de-ionized, it also serves as a solvent for the rinse.

Other than water, propylene glycol is the most common moisture-carrying vehicle used in the beauty industry. It has the ability to absorb moisture and act like a wetting agent. As well as being a common ingredient in the formulation of rinses, it is commonly used in mascara, hair straighteners, shaving lotions, mouthwashes, lipsticks, cold creams, emollients, makeup, and baby lotions.

FD&C and D&C pigments, acid dyes, and direct dyes are used as colorants in the instant rinses. The FD&C and D&C pigments, whether coal tar or petrochemical, are government certified as having a low incidence of allergic reaction. The remaining dyes have not been government certified, which means that the public must rely on industry standards of consumer safety.

Tartaric acid, citric acid, and phosphoric acid are all pH adjusters. Their addition creates an acid condition that increases substantivity (substantial adherence) to the hair.

Benzyl alcohol, SD alcohol, and isopropyl alcohol are used as solvents in instant rinses as well as perfumes. Benzyl alcohol has a faint sweet odor, but the product itself can be irritating and corrosive to the skin. The term SD alcohol covers a group of alcohols, all of which have been denatured. Denaturing alcohol refers to a process that makes the smell and taste so obnoxious that no one is likely to drink it. Isopropyl alcohol, added to achieve denaturing, works as a solvent and also serves as an antibacterial. It is used in many cosmetics, hand lotions, and after-shave lotions. Ingestion of isopropyl alcohol can cause headache, mental depression, nausea, vomiting, and coma. While it exhibits no toxicity on the surface of the skin, ingestion of approximately one ounce can prove fatal.

Ethyl cellulose, or hydroxyethylcellulose, is a binding, dispersing, and emulsifying agent made from wood pulp. It is often used over other similar chemicals because it is not susceptible to bacterial or fungal decomposition. Octoxynol is another chemical that can be used as an emulsifier in temporary rinses. It is a waxlike substance that is also utilized as a detergent and dispersing agent in hand creams, lotions, and lipsticks. Neither ethyl cellulose nor octoxynol have any known toxicity.

Butyl ester of PVM/MA copolymer is the abbreviated form of butyl ester of poly methyl vinyl ether, maleic acid. It is a plastic or resin that is also utilized in hair sprays, setting lotions, and serves as a thickener. Vinyl acetate and vinyl neodecanoate polymer fall within a major class of polymers that serves as a plasticizer in temporary rinses, as well as a resin in false nails and nail lacquer preparations. While inhalation of 300 parts per million of most vinyl by-products is toxic to man, neither butyl ester of PVM/MA copolymer, vinyl acetate or vinyl neodecanoate polymer has any known toxicity when applied to the skin within the formulation of a rinse.

Crotonic acid or beta-methacrylic acid is utilized in the manufacture of the resins that make up the composition of temporary rinses. It is found in clay, wood, and soil. Being found in nature, and the fact that it is used in the manufacture of vitamin A, makes crotonic acid appear to be a safe chemical, and in the proportions used in a temporary color rinse formula, it is safe. However, in its undiluted state, crotonic acid is a strong skin and mucous membrane irritant.

Aminomethylpropanol is added to emulsify and neutralize the above resins. Ammonia is also added for its ability to neutralize resins. However, a formulation with excessive ammonia may open the cuticle and cause a temporary rinse to deposit deeper than expected or desired.

Stearalkonium chloride, belonging to a large group of quaternary ammonium compounds, is commonly used in a variety of temporary colors for its preservative and germicidal properties. PEG 15 is a quaternary that helps condition the hair, making it easier to comb. All the quaternary ammonium compounds can be toxic at certain doses and concentrations.

Polyacrylamide is a white, solid, water-soluble polymer utilized as a thickening agent in rinses as well as in the manufacture of plastics used in nail polish. It is highly toxic and irritating to the skin. It can be absorbed through the unbroken skin. If contact is excessive, central nervous system paralysis may occur.

Safety

Temporary rinses are among the safest chemicals used in the cosmetology industry. The pH range of temporary color rinses is on the acid side of the scale, between 2.0 and 4.5. This low pH does not open the cuticle to allow for penetration of the large pigment molecule. The mixture simply sits on the outside of the hair shaft, causing no damage or chemical change in the structure of the hair.

Within the beauty industry temporary rinses are sometimes called certified rinses. This harbors the misconception that all the dyes and pigments used in these products are FDA certified. Many of the colorants are certified, but some are not. For this reason the bottle carries the FDA warning statement and the recommendation for a predisposition test.

INSTANT TEMPORARY RINSE COLOR CHART

EXPERIMENT INSTRUCTION SHEET

Objectives

To create a color chart of temporary rinses. To identify the level and tone of the rinse.

Directions

Select two rinses from each of the 10 levels of color—one warm and one cool. Apply rinse to a small piece of white cotton. Shape each into a neat little ball and glue in place at the appropriate color level. Label the cotton balls as to color name and tone of each rinse.

Materials Needed

- Instant temporary rinses
- Cotton

Level 1 Black   **Level 2 Dark brown**

_____   _____

_____   _____

Level 3 Medium brown   **Level 4 Light brown**

_____   _____

_____   _____

Level 5 Lightest brown   **Level 6 Dark blonde**

_____   _____

_____   _____

Level 7 Medium blonde   **Level 8 Light blonde**

_____   _____

_____   _____

Level 9 Very light blonde   **Level 10 Lightest blonde**

_____   _____

_____   _____

COLOR SHAMPOOS

Color shampoos are also known as highlighting shampoos. They are combinations of rinse and shampoo, which act similarly to temporary color rinses in that they give only slight color changes that are removed with plain shampooing. Color shampoos are used to highlight, impart slight color, and eliminate unwanted tones.

Chemical Composition

Color shampoos are formulated with noncertified and certified water-soluble dyes at the rate of 0.5 to 2.0 percent dyestuff, depending upon the desired hue, level, and saturation. The dye is dissolved in water and mixed with a shampoo detergent base such as amphoteric-2, triethanolamine or monoethanolamine lauryl sulphate. pH adjusters are added to create approximately a 5.0 to 6.5 acid absorption. A lower pH could result in an acid that, with vigorous massage, is strong enough to damage skin and eyes.

While regular shampoos list the number one ingredient as either de-ionized or purified water, color shampoos tend to list just plain water on their labels.

Trideceth is added to this formulation to improve resistance to moisture and oxidation. This chemical works as a binder, plasticizing agent, softener, and is a solvent also used in hair straighteners, hair tonics, protective creams, and baby products.

Lauramide DEA, a derivative of coconut oil, is added as a softener in cosmetic soaps and detergents as well as color shampoos. It has the ability to make large sudsy bubbles. Lauramide DEA can cause skin irritation.

Quaternium 19, derived from cellulose, is a film-former and binder that gives hair sheen. Glycol stearate is a combination of glycerine and alcohol utilized in cosmetics as a humectant. The formulation of a color shampoo containing quaternium 19 and glycol stearate helps to leave the hair soft and lustrous upon completion of the service.

Benzalkonium chloride is added for its germicidal effects. While incompatible with most detergents and soaps, it is soluble in water and alcohol; therefore, it is effective in a formulation of color shampoo that contains glycol or other forms of alcohol.

Hydrolyzed milk protein, milk protein processed into a simpler form for improved attachment to the hair shaft, also works to improve the finished appearance and condition of the hair.

Because marketing studies show that pleasant smelling products sell better than those that are not, fragrances such as phenethyl alcohol are added to give a floral scent. Phenethyl alcohol serves a dual purpose by also exhibiting preservative qualities. It has no known skin toxicity.

Safety

Color shampoos generally are considered safe. They may slightly dry and irritate some skin types, but most are classified as harmless. However, as with all coloring products, they carry the FDA safety warning and recommendation for a predisposition test due to the lack of government testing on such products.

COLOR SPRAYS

Temporary color sprays are applied from an aerosol can. They can be sprayed over the entire head of hair to create an even tone, such as a brown or auburn, but they are more popular for creating special and exotic effects.

Chemical Composition

Color sprays are most commonly formulated to be alcohol soluble. However, others are either water soluble or both oil and spirit soluble. Most color sprays are lacquer based, containing approximately .2 to .5 percent perfume and 99 percent alcohol.

Isopropyl alcohol, alcohol SDA 40, and propyl alcohol are used in a variety of combinations and amounts. These alcohols, manufactured by the fermentation of starch, sugar, and other carbohydrates, are widely used in cosmetics such as cold cream, after-shave lotions, face packs, hair lacquers, perfumes, shampoos, skin lotions, suntan lotions, and oils. Medicinally, alcohol is used as an external antiseptic, but it can dry both hair and skin when used to excess.

The small portion of the remaining formulation is generally a mixture of colorants, plastic resins, and solvents other than alcohol. Polyvinylpyrrolidone, PVP, and PVP/VA copolymer are all terms that indicate plastic resins or polymers, which are added to encourage the color to stick to the hair shaft. These ingredients are very controversial as used in the beauty industry. *(See section on Safety, page 33.)*

Vinyl acetate is formulated into the streaking sprays. Vinyl acetate is a resin from a major class of polymer materials widely used in plastics, synthetic fibers, and surface coatings. These materials are made from the reaction between acetylene and certain compounds such as alcohol, phenol, and animes. Inhalation of 300 parts per million is toxic to man.

A great variety of certified colorants are used in the sprays that give a natural color illusion. For example, FD&C red no. 3 is used at a concentration of approximately .1 percent to impart a warm auburn hue to medium brown hair. FD&C violet no. 1 in a .02 percent formulation adds ash blonde tones to bleached hair, and FD&C yellow no. 5 at the higher percent of .2 is used to impart golden highlights to medium brown hair.

Metallic powders, such as bronze powder, are used to create the gold and silver effects in streaking sprays. These metallic powders have been known to cause complications with future chemical services. The FD&C colorant used in these sprays is temporary, but metallic salts tend to coat the hair permanently. Thus the color may be completely removed from the hair, but upon repeated use the metallic salts may build up in the hair and react adversely with the application of a chemical service that incorporates either ammonia, hydrogen peroxide, or urea peroxide. The section on metallic hair coloring deals with this in depth.

Titanium dioxide is added in the formulation of sprays designed to create white streaks. Titanium dioxide is a white pigment with good covering and tinting power. It is also used in bath powders, depilatories, eyeliners, white eye shadows, antiperspirants, nail whites, face powders, protective creams, lipsticks, and hand lotions. No toxicity to man is known. In fact it is considered so safe for ingestion that sometimes it is used as the white pigment in candy and gum. However, in high concentrations the dust may cause lung damage.

Propylene glycol is added to the basic formula of color sprays to create streaking sprays. Propylene glycol is a clear, colorless liquid added as a moisture-carrying vehicle. It is inexpensive, but has received criticism because of reported allergic reactions.

Methylene chloride and dimethyl phthalate (phthalic esters) are used as solvents, to dissolve and disperse the contents of the container. Methylene chloride is a colorless gas that compresses into a liquid of pleasant odor and sweet taste. It is also used as an anesthetic in medicine. It can be absorbed through the pores of the skin, where it is converted into carbon monoxide. High levels of concentration are narcotic and cause stress in the cardiovascular system as well as damage to the kidneys, liver, and central nervous system.

Dimethyl phthalate is a colorless, aromatic oil that is also used as a solvent in calamine lotion and insect repellents. It is made from phthalic acid, which can be found naturally in some fungi. Dimethyl phthalate can be irritating to both skin and mucous membranes.

A glass marble is added to each can in the packaging. The concept is the same as aerosol spray paints. The glass marble is moved around in the can to discourage lumping and sediment settling.

The rub-off factor of this coloring product differs from manufacturer to manufacturer and from color to color within each line. Some suffer from excessive rub-off, leaving traces of color on combs, brushes, clothing, and pillowcases, while others are difficult to remove, even with shampooing.

Safety

Color sprays do not have a high incidence of allergic reaction and do not require a predisposition test. However, they do have other safety characteristics to consider. Inhalation of a concentrated amount can be harmful and even fatal. PVP or PVP/VA copolymer is an ingredient in almost all color sprays that is considered harmless when applied to the skin in solution form such as a rinse. However, when floating through the air this ingredient can enter through the mouth and nose. Concentrated doses of PVP from hair sprays have led to thesaurosis (a medical term indicating foreign bodies in the lung). Ingestion can damage lungs and kidneys. Modest intravenous doses in rats are believed responsible for the development of tumors.

The metallic salts in color sprays can build up after repeated use and cause an adverse reaction with future chemical services. These products are also extremely flammable, so they cannot be used around clients that are smoking.

COLOR MOUSSES, GELS, AND CREAMS

Color Mousses

Color mousses are one of the most contemporary ways to temporarily color the hair. They offer a wide array of colors that are fast and easy to apply. Color mousses serve many of the same purposes as temporary rinses. They can brighten, highlight, tone gray, disguise regrowth lines, and blend uneven color as well as create dramatic effects.

Color mousses stay put on the hair shaft. They do not drip, run, or blow off the hair when blow drying. This characteristic, and the fact that they do not appear to be a traditional hair color, makes them popular with men. They also give the hair body and volume. Some mousses have de-tangling and conditioning abilities.

Chemical Composition

The first ingredient listed in most mousses is water. A second common ingredient is either SD alcohol or isopropyl alcohol, also known as isopropanol. The letters "SD" before alcohol are an abbreviation for "specially denatured," indicating in this instance that a poison has been added to make the alcohol unfit for consumption. Isopropyl alcohol is prepared from propylene, which is obtained from petroleum. Isopropyl alcohol is also used in body rubs, hand lotions, after-shave lotions, antifreeze, and shellac.

While it has no known toxicity on the skin, ingestion or inhalation of large quantities of the vapor may cause headache, dizziness, nausea, vomiting, mental depression, and coma. Approximately one fluid ounce is fatal when ingested.

Butane, isobutane, and propane are used in color mousses as a propellant or aerosol. Large doses of butane can lead to asphyxiation, but the immediate danger is of fire and explosion. Propane, a gas that is heavier than air, is also used as a fuel and a refrigerant. In aerosol cans it also serves as an aerator. Both butane and propane may be narcotic in large doses. Isobutane is a derivative of natural gas.

One or more of the polyquaternium compounds or PEG-2 oleamonium chloride can be found on the ingredient listing of most mousses. These chemicals are a variety of synthetic derivatives used as preservatives, surfactants, antiseptics, and germicides that can irritate the skin, eyes, and mucous membranes. Ingestion of any quaternium compound can be toxic and even fatal if the dose and concentration are great enough.

Dimethicone copolyol, sometimes listed as just dimethicone, is a silicone oil with very low toxicity that is used as a skin protectant. It is derived from silica. This natural ingredient, found in 12 percent of all rocks, is a coloring agent.

Citric acid (vitamin C) is added not only for its kindness to skin through its ability to balance an alkali solution, but for its ability to close the cuticle layer of the hair and skin. This helps to prevent unwanted penetration of the color molecules.

Small amounts of nonoxynol are commonly added to the formulation to help the product spread. Nonoxynol is nontoxic and used in many cosmetic products.

Fragrance, of course, is added to make the product pleasant to use. A variety of acid dyes and colorants taken from the FD&C approved list are used in color mousses, gels, and creams. A few contain small amounts of metallic salts.

Color Gels and Creams

The color gels and creams are available in a variety of shades, some natural, others wild and vibrant. These colors are designed to shampoo completely out, but because they tend to be hues of intense saturation, they may stain porous, bleached, or very dry hair.

Chemical Composition

Typically, water is the number one ingredient of these products, followed by either PVP/VA or isopropyl alcohol. PVP/VA is a copolymer used in color creams and gels as a setting agent that provides a flexible film with low incidence of tackiness. Isopropyl alcohol is the same ingredient used in color mousses as an antibacterial, solvent, and denaturant. Both ingredients are used just as they are in color mousses and come with the same safety and toxicity characteristics.

Dimethyl phthalate is a colorless, aromatic oil, insoluble in water, that is added as a solvent. It is a common ingredient in insect repellent and calamine lotion.

Acrylates, such as ammonium acrylates copolymer, thicken gels. This ingredient is a salt or ester of acrylic acid, also used in nail polish, that can be a skin irritant.

Cocamidopropyl betaine, a derivative of coconut oil, is a white, semisolid, highly saturated fat that is also used in the manufacture of baby soaps, shampoos, shaving lathers, and massage creams. It is stable when exposed to air and helps to give gels and creams spreadability. Generally considered safe, in strong concentrates cocamidopropyl betaine may irritate the skin enough to cause rashes.

Methylparaben (small, odorless, colorless crystals) and propylparaben (esters of p-hydroxybenzoic acid) are widely used preservatives and bactericides. They are nontoxic in small amounts but can cause allergic reactions on the skin.

DMDM hydantoin is also used for its preservative actions in many cosmetics. It is a compound that slowly liberates formaldehyde. Formaldehyde in strong concentrations is a chemical that kills living tissue. Many consumer agencies have fought unsuccessfully to have it removed from all cosmetics.

Hydroxyethylcellulose works as a binding, dispersing, and emulsifying agent in color gels, color creams, and many other cosmetics. It is made from wood pulp or cotton. It has no known toxicity.

To create the desired hue, level, and saturation the manufacturers use a variety of pigments, FD&C, and D&C colors. Titanium dioxide, the white pigment used in candy, gum, and marking ink, also appears regularly on the ingredients list.

Iron oxides, such as those used in color crayons, are commonly used. They may be any of several natural or synthetic oxides of iron (combination of iron and oxygen), varying in color from red to brown, black to yellow, depending upon the purity and the amount of water added.

Safety of Color Mousses, Gels, and Creams

Repeated use of iron oxides can cause complications with future chemical treatments because, as the color shampoos out, the iron oxide, like any metallic salt, remains permanently affixed to the shaft. The other colorants used are of low toxicity and allergic reaction so no predisposition test is required by the FDA. However, direct inhalation or ingestion of these products can cause brain damage or even death. Formaldehyde has been under scrutiny for years. However, it has not been rated as a "significant" health risk in the small quantities used in these products.

HAIR COLOR CRAYONS

The primary purpose of hair color crayons is to blend regrowth between retouches. They are manufactured in stick form and in a small variety of colors. This form of coloring was popular in the mid-1900's.

Chemical Composition

One of the primary ingredients in color crayons is tea-stearate, which is a combination of triethanolamine and stearic acid. The purpose of this compound is to absorb moisture. Tea-stearate is cream colored but turns brown on exposure to air. It is also used in shaving creams, baby preparations, mascaras, fragrances, liquid makeups, cleansing and foundation creams, hair lacquers, and protective creams.

The hair crayon has a wax base, made of a combination of two or more of the following waxes: paraffin, beeswax, or microcrystalline wax. Paraffin is an odorless, greasy product obtained from the distillate of wood, coal, petroleum, or shale oil.

This white or colorless wax serves as a base in many formulations of lipsticks, eyebrow pencils, protective creams, liquefying creams, and mascaras.

Beeswax from virgin bees is yellowish white and used primarily as an emulsifier in cosmetics such as emollient creams, brilliantine hairdressings, cold creams, wax depilatories, nail whiteners, rouges, mascaras, and protective creams.

Microcrystalline wax is a plastic material obtained from petroleum. It differs from paraffin waxes in structure and action in that it is composed of much finer crystals that can only be detected under a microscope. As well, the viscosity and melting point are higher in the microcrystalline waxes than the paraffins. Cake cosmetics and nail polishes also utilize microcrystalline wax in their formulations.

A variety of the same dyestuffs used in other temporary colors are used in this simple formulation to create the different shades of color crayons. While not all are FDA certified, this product does not carry the government warning label requiring a predisposition test.

Ultramarine blue, which is added to the formulation to create the black color crayon, has a most interesting background. This blue occurs naturally in the mineral lapis lazuli, which is still widely used today in the making of gemstone jewelry. Originally the color was obtained from the grinding of the stone. However, it is now produced synthetically. Cosmetically, it is also used in eye shadow, mascara, and face powder, as well as serving as a bluing in laundry products and a coloring of tiles.

Neither lapis lazuli nor its synthetic replacement have shown toxicity when used on the surface of the skin. However, workmen handling the powdered product suffer from lung and nose disorders such as ulceration and perforation of the septum (the dividing wall of the nose).

Most colorants used in color crayons are safe and completely compatible with future chemical services. However, some hair crayons use metallic salts such as iron oxides and titanium dioxide in their formulation to increase color fastness.

Safety

All three waxes, paraffin, beeswax, and microcrystalline wax, are nontoxic and considered harmless. However, eczemas as well as precancerous and cancerous conditions have been traced to impurities in paraffin. The wax base of color crayons retards the absorption of liquids and thereby makes it necessary to completely remove the coloring from the hair before the next chemical service.

The metallic salts in this color, just as in other colors, can lead to complications in subsequent chemical services. Discoloration, damage, and even breakage of the hair strands have been known to occur from metallic salts residue.

MASCARA

Mascara crosses the line between a hair coloring and makeup product. It is considered a temporary hair coloring because it temporarily colors the hair of the eyelashes with a variety of neutral shades—brown and black—as well as the colors of an artist's palette—blue, violet, and teal, just to name a few. Mascara gives the illusion of density and length to the lashes.

The trend setting ancient Egyptians led the way with the creation of mascara. The early formula was known as Kohol or Kohl. It was a mixture of antimony sulphide, lead sulfur, copper oxide, and magnesium oxide mixed with oil and applied with a stick to the eyebrows and eyelashes. Advanced technology has brought present day consumers a much safer formulation.

Chemical Composition

Cake mascara is made of ethanolamine soap, which is only mildly alkaline and has a low incidence of irritation, blended with wax and molded into a bar. Beeswax, carnauba wax, and spermaceti are three of the most commonly used because of their compatibility with soap.

Silicone oils are added to increase the products' resistance to moisture. Glyceryl monostearate is a binding material that helps form a smooth paste when the cake is dampened for application.

Cream mascara has lost popularity, but it is still required in many states by the State Board of Cosmetology because of its sanitary method of application. The cream is packaged in a small tube and squeezed out onto a clean applicator brush. Cream mascara has good lasting properties that are usually prepared from an emulsion base of thiethanolamine stearate, containing about 5 percent of polyvinyl alcohol or a film-forming resin such as polyvinyl acetate, or a film-forming copolymer. Beeswax is often added primarily as an emulsifier.

Many wand mascaras are formulated with the new long-lasting polymer products. These are plastic-based fixatives that help mascara stay put until it is time to take it off. They also contain water, wax, coloring agents, thickeners, film-formers, and preservatives. Some contain up to 5 percent rayon or nylon fibers to build up or thicken the lashes.

Over the last decade, mascara has become less temporary than in the past. A true temporary color can be removed with soap or shampoo. Most manufacturers today produce a mascara that requires a petroleum or solvent based cleanser to remove all traces of color.

The black shades, still the most popular in mascaras, are prepared with a cosmetic grade of carbon in a range of particle sizes. For the brown and brownish-black hues the black carbon is blended with a suitable cosmetic brown oxide. Ultramarine blue is used with carbon black to create a blue-black shade. Chromium oxide and hydrated chromium oxide are used for the brilliant blue-greens.

Perfume is an unnecessary ingredient in mascara, yet some manufacturers do add a rose-type perfume of a non-sensitizing and nonirritating type.

Safety

Even though some mascaras make the eyes water and burn, the composition of mascara is balanced and controlled enough to be considered safe. The danger lies in contamination of a product that is used so close to sensitive mucous membranes and in the possibility of poking the eye with the applicator. Reports have also been recorded of waterproof mascaras scratching when they get in the eye rather than merely dissolving as water soluble mascaras do.

COLOR POWDERS

Color powders are brushed or sprinkled on to create temporary streaks or tones to the hair. Some contain metallic salts while others do not. However, color powder is generally applied to dry hair so that the metallic salts do not adhere to a softened cuticle. Color powders comprise a minute portion of the hair color market and are produced by only a few companies.

Safety

Color powders are generally safe for use, having little toxicity or known allergic reaction. However, they can be extremely irritating to the mucous membranes of the eye and, if the particles are sharp, can scratch the eye.

3
Semipermanent Hair Coloring

Semipermanent colors are commercially known by a variety of names: *monthly rinses, semipermanent tints,* and *semipermanent rinses.* The term "monthly rinse" indicates that this product is designed to last approximately one month. "Semipermanent tint" infers color that is partly but not completely permanent. "Semipermanent rinse" refers to the ability to gradually rinse completely out of the hair with shampooing. The regular use of three different terms to indicate the same color product may be confusing to the beginning colorist. However, the terms simply describe different aspects of the same coloring product.

Two basic classifications of semipermanent color are currently available: *traditional* and *polymer.* They are designed to meet a variety of needs: to enhance natural hair color, tone pre-lightened hair, enhance and cover gray, and to create fashion colors. Most semipermanent colors are formulated for use on natural hair, a smaller number are designed for tinted or bleached hair, and an even smaller group are the polymer colors that can have either a natural appearance or may be bold and bright.

Semipermanent rinses are deposition colors. They deposit color in the cortex layer of the hair as well as coating the shaft. They are considered "self-penetrating" for two reasons. The first reason is that semipermanent colors utilize basic dyes and direct dyes rather than pigments that must be mixed with hydrogen peroxide for color development. The second reason is that this formulation contains a mild oxidizer to open the cuticle and allow penetration.

This mild oxidizer allows semipermanent colors to add warmth, coolness, or depth, but does not offer the power to substantially lift or lighten. The use of a white or silvery tone on either bleached or naturally gray hair may create a lightening effect. However, the chemical composition of the product does not allow sufficient diffusion of melanin to create any appreciable change to a lighter level. The illusion of lightening is achieved by camouflaging or neutralizing the desired yellow.

Like temporary colors, semipermanent colors provide an excellent introduction to color. The client may "try out" a color before committing to a permanent tint. A large variety of darkening, high-fashion, and toning colors are available for experimentation or regular use.

Semipermanent colors are economical to use in that most spread very easily, making the standard application only two ounces of product. However, when mixing colors to achieve the desired shade, waste can occur because the opened, half-used bottles of traditional semipermanent colors begin to lose their potency after 30 days.

39

TRADITIONAL SEMIPERMANENT COLORS

Traditional semipermanent colors have several distinct differences from temporary and permanent colors. They last longer than temporary colors and do not rub off. They also are easy to use, requiring no retouch application, just reapplication. Because semipermanent colors make no significant permanent changes in the structure of the hair, they are less damaging. Some brands even give a conditioning effect. They are excellent for toning bleached hair that is too weak or porous to accept another peroxide treatment and for use on hair that is exceptionally fine or damaged from permanent wave or relaxer services.

However, discoloration and off-tones can result from the mildness and inability of semipermanent colors to make changes in the composition of the hair. A green cast on gray, white, and blonde hair when coloring to a brown shade is one example of this. The color brown is created by pigment that reflects red, yellow, and blue light waves. The molecules that reflect blue light rays are larger in size and thus have more difficulty penetrating the cuticle. Therefore, it is common for the manufacturer to add a greater percentage of the blue pigment to achieve sufficient deposition. Porous hair can absorb too many blue molecules and a variety of off-tones result depending upon the natural color of the hair. If the residual shade is yellow, a green off-tone commonly results. Turquoise results if the residual shade was blue-gray and plain blue if the hair was white.

Excessive red highlights are another problem that can occur with semipermanent colors. The molecules reflecting red light rays are smaller, penetrate deeper, and thus tend to remain in the cortex longer than the blue and gray colors. This results in the pigment molecules being removed at different rates, leaving behind and exposing the red tones.

Excessive red can also be caused by the activators within the product. Ammonia, thio, urea peroxide, sodium perborate, and alkalies all affect the natural pigment of the hair. They each cause a slight diffusion of melanin that results in the reflection of more red and orange light rays.

All of these color problems can be solved with one or more of the following methods. The first solution is to utilize the Chromatic Circle and the neutralization concept to correct the unwanted tones. The second method is to switch the client to another brand of semipermanent color. If this does not solve the problem, switching to a permanent tint may be necessary.

Occasionally, a semipermanent color will grab darker on the ends than on the rest of the shaft. This occurs when the ends are over-porous. To blend the color, use a "retouch application" rather than the "standard reapplication" method generally done.

Color Selection

The addition of artificial color molecules to the natural pigment of the hair shaft will create a color that is darker than the sample on the color chart. Most color charts show approximately the color that will be achieved on white hair. This color is to be used as a guide to estimate the color results when it is applied to natural hair.

The natural hair color must be considered as half the formula. Think of it as "1/2 artificial color and 1/2 natural color." Semipermanent colors lack the strong oxidizers necessary to lift; therefore they deposit color and do no substantial lifting. Think back to the laws of saturation and remember that color applied on top of color makes a darker color.

The following steps, used in conjunction with the manufacturer's color chart, offer a guide to selecting the correct hue with which to perform a test strand:

1. On solid hair (no gray) select a level of color that is two levels lighter than the desired shade. (For gray coverage, see chart in the section titled *Gray and White Hair on page 125.*)
2. Due to the absorption of light, the use of an ash or cool shade will create a color that the eye interprets as darker than if a warm shade is applied.
3. Due to the reflection of light, the warm colors will appear shinier.

Chemical Composition

Traditional semipermanent colors are formulated with pigment molecules that are smaller than those of the temporary colors but larger than those of the permanent tints. The chemical composition of semipermanent colors falls within the approximate pH range of 8.0-9.0, thus causing an alkaline reaction on the hair. The alkali swells the cuticle, opening imbrications, allowing the molecules to enter the cortex. However, this solution is mildly alkaline, which causes limited swelling and opening. Only a small number of these medium-sized molecules enter and remain in the cortex, but a stronger alkali solution would weaken the hair strands, causing structural damage and excessive penetration of the color.

The pigment molecules are trapped within the cortical layer of the shaft as the hair shrinks back toward normal during the rinsing step of the service. A neutral or slightly acid after-rinse helps to close the imbrications and hold the pigment molecules within the cortex. However, even the mild swelling that occurs with shampooing allows some of the color to fade.

Some formulations use salt bonds to improve color fastness. This formulation allows a lower pH of 7.0-8.0 and affects the condition of the hair less than the product with a higher pH.

Other manufacturers use a weakened ammonium thioglycolate in their semipermanent colors. Thio has the ability to separate keratin and allow more pigment to pass into the cortex. Therefore, the hair must be handled carefully until it is dry. As the hair dries, it undergoes atmospheric (air) oxidation and the bonds are reformed. However, thio also causes the breaking of S-bonds and the weakening of the hair structure. With this type of semipermanent color an acid rinse is recommended to neutralize the alkali.

A typical semipermanent formula is:

- Water—50 percent or more
- Surfactants—up to 10 percent
- Perfumes—up to 10 percent
- Solvents—up to 6 percent
- Color pigments—up to 5 percent
- Thickeners—up to 5 percent
- pH balancers—up to 5 percent
- Stabilizers—approximately .1 percent

Most of the dyes used in semipermanent colors are basic dyes and in particular a sub-category known as nitro-dyes. The prefix, nitro, denotes one atom of nitrogen and two of oxygen. It also denotes a class of dyes derived from coal tars.

Listed below is a group of nitro-dyes related to coal tar that are common to most semipermanent home and professional dyes:

- 3-nitro-n-hydroxyethyl-p-phenylenediamine
- n,n^1-dimethyl-n-hydroxyethyl-3-nitro-p-phenylenediamine
- 2-nitro-5-glyceryl-methylaniline
- 3-nitro-p-hydroxyethylaminophenol

Aminophenol is used in semipermanent hair colors that have dyeing action only when exposed to oxygen. This chemical, discovered in London in 1854, is derived from phenol, which is obtained from coal tar. Aminophenol is an aromatic, colorless crystal that is also known as:

- o-aminophenol
- m-aminophenol
- 4-amino-2-nitrophenol
- p-aminophenol HCl
- p-aminophenol
- 2-amino-5-nitrophenol
- 2-amino-6-chloro-4-nitrophenol

Phenylenediamine, also used in oxidation colors, is sometimes known commercially as amino dye, para dye, peroxide dye, or just plain PPD. Chemically it is a developed dye. It was first used in 1890 to dye furs and feathers. It is available in approximately 30 shades and is used as an intermediate in coal tar dyes. The final color is achieved by oxidation of the color that penetrates the hair shaft. Butoxyethanol, or butyl cellosolve, is an ingredient added as a solvent for resins, grease, oil, and albumin (a protein found in egg white). It helps to disperse the semipermanent color and dissolve grease, oil, and dirt from the shaft so that the color can penetrate.

Polyglyceryl-2-oleyl ether is an organic compound made from glycerin polymers and oleyl alcohol. It too is a solvent, but it also works as a humectant that keeps the product from drying out.

Isopropanol and benzyl alcohol can be combined for use as a solvent in semipermanent color. The isopropanol alcohol also works as an antibacterial agent and a denaturant. Produced from petroleum, isopropanol is a common ingredient in hand lotions, after-shave lotions, and antifreeze. Benzyl alcohol is a pure alcohol also used as a solvent in perfumes.

One of the fragrances used in semipermanent colors is "tall oil" or "liquid rosin." "Tall" is Swedish for "pine." Tall oil is used to scent shampoos, soaps, and varnishes as well. It also doubles as a fungicide and a cutting oil.

Tallow amide is a compound made from the fatty tissue of cattle in North America. It is white and generally harder than grease. It may cause eczema and blackheads on the skin. Amide on the end of tallow indicates that a derivative of ammonia is added to this compound. The purpose of the addition of "amides" is to raise the pH and soften and open the cuticle of the hair shaft.

Aminomethyl propanol is an alcohol made from nitrogen compounds. It serves as an emulsifier in semipermanent colors but is also used in cosmetic creams and lotions.

Coconut diethanolamine is a foaming agent that controls distribution of the colorant. It is also added for its ability to act as a solvent and emulsifier.

Hydrophilic colloids, such as methyl cellulose, carbopol, or a natural gum, are added to thicken the viscosity. These substances are suspended in water.

Hydroxyethylcellulose or ethylcellulose works in a manner similar to the coconut diethanolamine as a dispersing and emulsifying agent and similar to the hydrophilic colloids as a thickening agent. It also serves as a diluent in semipermanent colors, nail polishes, and many other color additive mixtures.

Cocomide DEA, derived from coconut oil, assists with foaming. It is also used in the manufacture of shampoos, soaps, and massage creams.

Lauric acid, or dodecanoic acid, also made from coconut oil, is used because of its foaming properties and ability to adjust pH. It has a slight odor of bay and makes large luxurious bubbles in soap. It can be a mild irritant.

Citric acid, derived from citrus fruit, is one of the most commonly used acid balancing agents in semipermanent colors as well as many other cosmetics. It also acts as a foam inhibitor, plasticizer, and preservative. Citric acid is used in skin fresheners, eye lotions, hair rinses, and in a sugar and water solution as a cool summer drink.

Methyl paraben is a widely used preservative. It is effective in hair colorings because of its stability over a wide acid/alkalinity range. Propylparaben, butylparaben, and ethylparaben are esters of p-hydroxybenzoic acid. They are all widely used in the beauty industry as preservatives. Other products in which they are utilized are shampoos, wave sets, eye lotions, beauty masks, baby preparations, foundation creams, and dentifrices. These esters are used medicinally to treat fungus infections. While they can cause contact dermatitis, they are low in toxicity and active in all pH ranges: alkaline, neutral, acid.

Semipermanent rinses have some cation-active properties and, therefore, are absorbed to some extent by the hair fiber. Synthetic detergents consisting of quaternary ammonium compounds with carbon and nitrogen are added to assist with absorption, spreadability, and preservation of the product.

Activators

Many semipermanent colors are used just as they pour from the bottle. However, others require the mixing of an activator prior to application. This activator is an oxidant that helps to swell the cortex and open the cuticle for color penetration. This mild oxidizer also develops the color pigments within the formula. The active ingredient in these activators is generally either urea peroxide, sodium perborate, or thioglycolic acid.

Urea peroxide is a white crystal oxidant packaged in powder form to be added to semipermanent colors. It promotes oxygen release and the evolution of ammonia. The package should be stored in a dry cool area or it may begin to oxidize in the container. Urea peroxide powder must be handled carefully as it can cause severe eye and skin irritation. Ingestion may cause bleeding in the mouth and swelling of the esophagus.

Sodium perborate is a white crystalline salt that is classified as a catalyst when used with semipermanent colors. Highly alkaline, the compound is irritating to both the skin and mucous membranes. It must be kept dry, as any moisture will allow it to activate.

Thioglycolic acid, while better known for its role in permanent waving, sometimes can be found on the ingredient list of either the activator or the semipermanent color itself.

Color Balance Crystal

Some semipermanent colors include a color balancer in the packaging. This crystal need be added only if the semipermanent color is to be applied immediately following the removal of a lightening or bleaching product.

The color balance crystal contains only one ingredient, sodium erythorbate. Sodium erythorbate is an odorless, white crystal used as an antioxidant. It stops the residual oxidation that occurs on the hair shaft until the normal pH is completely restored.

After-Rinse

Some semipermanent colors come packaged with an "after-rinse." This rinse is acid balanced to close the cuticle and trap within it the color molecules. This helps to prevent fading to a lighter color as well as fading off-tone. The chemical composition of the after-rinse is designed to leave the hair soft, pliable, and easy to comb.

The main ingredient in the after-rinse packet is water. Citric acid is included to lower the pH of the solution and thus restore the acid balance of the hair shaft after the alkaline reaction of the semipermanent color.

Cetearyl alcohol, stearyl alcohol, and hydroxyethylcellulose all moisturize and lubricate the hair strand. Ceteth-2 is a compound of derivatives of cetyl, lauryl, stearyl, and oleyl alcohols that makes the rinse spread easily on the hair and helps create a surface on which the comb will easily glide.

Stearalkonium chloride, dicetyldimonium chloride, and quaternium-26 are quaternary ammonium compounds that are added as preservatives. The last ingredients generally are a light fragrance and a little certified vegetable color to make the rinse look and smell pretty.

Safety

The probable lethal dose of any semipermanent color for a 10 kg./21 lb. child is at least five ounces of this untasty solution. Therefore, it is unlikely that a child, and unthinkable that an adult, would drink enough for it to be fatal. Even though several of the ingredients listed above can lead to a variety of diseases and disorders, the product is classified as nontoxic.

Ingestion or inhalation of large quantities of the vapor of the ingredient isopropanol alcohol may cause headache, dizziness, mental depression, vomiting, and coma. Benzyl alcohol is much less toxic; however, it can be irritating and corrosive to the skin and mucous membranes.

The coal tar products, the aniline derivative and nitro-amino dyes, within the formulation of semipermanent colors can cause mild to violent allergic reactions. In its mildest form, the allergic reaction manifests itself in itching that can be treated with a vinegar or other acid rinse. More severe reactions include swelling, nausea, vomiting, dizziness, fever, coma, and heart failure. The possibility of these violent reactions makes the predisposition test, as required by the Federal Food, Drug, and Cosmetic Act, an important prerequisite for every semipermanent color service. While European regulations will not allow PPD in their products, the United States is still in the process of proving or disproving the increased risk of cancer with use of this product.

The paraben derivatives, as used to preserve traditional semipermanent colors, are classified as nonirritating, non-sensitizing, and nonpoisonous. Although most have been known to cause some allergic reactions and contact dermatitis, they are considered less toxic than some other commonly used preservatives.

LEVEL 8—SEMIPERMANENT COLOR RESULTS COMPARISON

EXPERIMENT INSTRUCTION SHEET

Objectives

To observe and document the results of application of the same blonde semipermanent color on four different levels of natural hair color. To gain experience working with semipermanent colors.

Hair Swatches Needed

4 virgin hair swatches of the following color levels:
- Level 8-9
- Level 5-6
- Level 2-3
- Salt and pepper

Labeling Hair Swatches

Label each swatch with the color to be used.

Materials Needed

- One level 8 semipermanent color product
- Plastic bags

Color Selection and Formulation

1. Follow manufacturer's recommended directions as to whether or not to pre-shampoo.
2. Select one level 8 shade and mix approximately 1 tablespoon of product following the manufacturer's recommended directions.

Procedure

1. If the manufacturer recommends covering the hair with a plastic bag during processing, place the swatches in a plastic bag to simulate this step.
2. Process at room temperature for 40 minutes.
3. Refer to the manufacturer's recommended directions as to whether or not to shampoo.
4. Rinse thoroughly. Continue to rinse and work the water through the hair for several minutes after the water rinses clean.
5. Dry and examine color results.
6. Mount swatches on the *Experiment Results Sheet on page R-3*.
7. Label each swatch with timing and formula used.
8. Answer *Review Questions on page R-5*.

LEVEL 5-6—AUBURN SEMIPERMANENT COLOR RESULTS COMPARISON

EXPERIMENT INSTRUCTION SHEET

Objectives

To observe results of application of the same auburn semipermanent color on four different levels of natural hair color. To gain experience working with semipermanent colors.

Hair Swatches Needed

4 virgin hair swatches of the following color levels:
- Level 8-9
- Level 5-6
- Level 2-3
- Salt and pepper

Labeling Hair Swatches

Label each swatch with the color to be used.

Materials Needed

- One level 5-6 auburn semipermanent color product
- Plastic bags

Color Selection and Formulation

1. Follow manufacturer's recommended directions as to whether or not to pre-shampoo.
2. Select one level 5-6 auburn shade and mix approximately 1 tablespoon of product following the manufacturer's recommended directions.

Procedure

1. If the manufacturer recommends covering the hair with a plastic bag during processing, place the swatches in a plastic bag to simulate this step.
2. Process at room temperature for 40 minutes.
3. Refer to the manufacturer's recommended directions as to whether or not to shampoo.
4. Rinse thoroughly. Continue to rinse and work the water through the hair for several minutes after the water rinses clean.
5. Dry and examine color results.
6. Mount swatches on the *Experiment Results Sheet on page R-7*.
7. Label each swatch with timing and formula used.
8. Answer *Review Questions on page R-9*.

LEVEL 3—SEMIPERMANENT COLOR RESULTS COMPARISON

EXPERIMENT INSTRUCTION SHEET

Objectives

To observe and document results of application of the same brown semipermanent color on four different levels of natural hair color. To gain experience working with semipermanent colors.

Hair Swatches Needed

4 virgin hair swatches of the following color levels:
- Level 8-9
- Level 5-6
- Level 2-3
- Salt and pepper

Labeling Hair Swatches

Label each swatch with the color to be used.

Materials Needed

- One level 3 semipermanent color product
- Plastic bags

Color Selection and Formulation

1. Follow manufacturer's recommended directions as to whether or not to pre-shampoo.
2. Select one level 3 shade and mix approximately 1 tablespoon of product following the manufacturer's recommended directions.

Procedure

1. If the manufacturer recommends covering the hair with a plastic bag during processing, place the swatches in a plastic bag to simulate this step.
2. Process at room temperature for 40 minutes.
3. Refer to the manufacturer's recommended directions as to whether or not to shampoo.
4. Rinse thoroughly. Continue to rinse and work the water through the hair for several minutes after the water rinses clean.
5. Dry and examine color results.
6. Mount swatches on the *Experiment Results Sheet on page R-11.*
7. Label each swatch with timing and formula used.
8. Answer *Review Questions on page R-13.*

LEVEL 1—SEMIPERMANENT COLOR RESULTS COMPARISON

EXPERIMENT INSTRUCTION SHEET

Objectives

To observe and document results of application of the same black semipermanent color on four different levels of natural hair color. To gain experience working with semipermanent colors.

Hair Swatches Needed

4 virgin hair swatches of the following color levels:
- Level 8-9
- Level 5-6
- Level 2-3
- Salt and pepper

Labeling Hair Swatches

Label each swatch with the color to be used.

Materials Needed

- One level 1 semipermanent color product
- Plastic bags

Color Selection and Formulation

1. Follow manufacturer's recommended directions as to whether or not to pre-shampoo.
2. Select one level 1 shade and mix approximately 1 tablespoon of product following the manufacturer's recommended directions.

Procedure

1. If the manufacturer recommends covering the hair with a plastic bag during processing, place the swatches in a plastic bag to simulate this step.
2. Process at room temperature for 40 minutes.
3. Refer to the manufacturer's recommended directions as to whether or not to shampoo.
4. Rinse thoroughly. Continue to rinse and work the water through the hair for several minutes after the water rinses clean.
5. Dry and examine color results.
6. Mount swatches on the *Experiment Results Sheet on page R-15.*
7. Label each swatch with timing and formula used.
8. Answer *Review Questions on page R-17.*

SEMIPERMANENT HAIR COLOR BRAND COMPARISON

EXPERIMENT INSTRUCTION SHEET

Objectives

To compare color results between different brands of semipermanent colors. To experience the mixing directions of different brands of this type of color.

Hair Swatches Needed

6 virgin hair swatches of the following color levels:

- 2 swatches of level 8-9 from the same head cutting
- 2 swatches of level 5-6 from the same head cutting
- 2 swatches of level 2-3 from the same head cutting

Labeling Hair Swatches

Label level 8-9 swatch with the color name and brand to be used. Label the second level 8-9 swatch with the color name and brand of the second product to be used. Continue with remaining swatches.

Materials Needed

- Level 7-8 semipermanent color—two different brands
- Level 4-5 semipermanent color—two different brands
- Level 1-2 semipermanent color—two different brands
- Any activators or rinses that accompany the particular brands selected for this experiment
- Plastic bags

Color Selection and Formulation

1. Select two different brands of semipermanent colors to work with.
2. Read manufacturer's recommended directions to determine if swatches must be pre-shampooed.
3. Following the individual manufacturer's recommended directions, mix approximately 1 tablespoon of each product.

Procedure

1. Thoroughly saturate each swatch with appropriate product.
2. If the manufacturer recommends covering the hair with a plastic bag during processing, place the swatches in a plastic bag to simulate this step.
3. Process at room temperature for 40 minutes.
4. Refer to the manufacturer's recommended directions as to whether to shampoo or not.
5. Rinse thoroughly. Continue to rinse and work the water through the hair for several minutes after the water rinses clean.
6. Dry and examine color results.
7. Mount swatches on *Experiment Results Sheet on pages R-19 and R-21.*
8. Answer *Review Questions on page R-23.*

POLYMER SEMIPERMANENT COLORS

The polymer colors are classified as semipermanent colors because they use direct, disperse, and certified dyes that require no oxidation process or the addition of an oxidizer for color development. However, they are distinctly different from traditional semipermanent colors in color results, color fastness, and chemical composition.

Color Selection

The polymer semipermanent colors were originally available in only highly saturated primary and secondary colors that added a high-fashion accent to natural hair color. They are currently available in more "natural" shades. The polymers are designed to coat and penetrate the shaft, creating translucent shine and accent hues rather than complete coverage of the natural color.

The color fastness or staying power of the polymer colors differs from traditional semipermanent colors. The polymer colors are advertised as colors that are removed gradually by shampooing. However, in many cases colorists have found this not to be true.

A polymer is a substance or product consisting of long-chain structural units created from the combining of many small molecules (monomers). These chains have tensile strength, elasticity, and hardness. Other examples of polymers are vinyl, plastic, rubber, and human tissue. The long-chain structure of the polymer actually inhibits its penetration of the cuticle and its ability to adhere to the keratin of the hair shaft. However, the dyes in polymer colors are extremely concentrated so that regardless of the long-chain structure, the color becomes well fixed to the hair.

Heat is a key factor in the staying power of the polymer colors. The higher the heat and the longer the processing time, the deeper the color penetration and the greater the color fastness. As a general rule, a polymer color that is applied for less than 25 minutes with moderate heat will behave like a semipermanent color. A polymer processed for 30 minutes or more with maximum heat penetrates deeply and attaches itself within the cortex in a manner that is as permanent as an oxidizing tint. This is how the polymer color often comes to act like a permanent color in staying power even though it utilizes no oxidizer.

Polymer colors have been known to become so well attached to the structure of the hair shaft that even bleaches or dye solvents prepared with hydrogen peroxide will not remove them. Salon experience has shown that often the natural pigment can be completely diffused and taken through all 7 stages of lightening while the polymer color, although lightened, is still apparent.

Regardless of the extensiveness of the experience of the colorist, performing a test strand is the most professional method of color selection. Both the color results and fastness of polymer colors are unique to this product. Therefore, a test strand is doubly important.

Polymers have no lifting or bleaching capabilities; therefore it is necessary only to concentrate on deposition. The natural melanin within the hair shaft will not be changed by this type of coloring. The color achieved will be the direct result of the addition of the polymer pigment to the natural pigment of the shaft.

Before selecting the shade of polymer to be used, analyze the natural level and tone of the hair. During the client consultation, determine if the objective is to neutralize, accent, or overpower the existing hue. When using the Artist's Concept of the Laws of Color to determine which shade will best achieve the desired tone, keep in mind that most shades of this product are highly saturated.

The level of depth and the degree of saturation achieved with a polymer color are determined by the length of time the hair is processed under heat. The longer the processing time and the higher the temperature, the deeper and longer lasting the color.

Polymer colors are sometimes added to the neutralizing solution after a permanent wave. The softened physical structure and temporarily unstable chemical composition of the hair allows for permanent deposition without the use of heat.

The bright primary hues are difficult to achieve on black hair. To achieve more deposition in dark hair, the polymer colors can be used immediately after a relaxing service. Again the softened state of the shaft allows for more deposition than can be achieved on non-chemically treated hair.

The following chart will assist in color selection of the polymer colors. It should be used as a cross reference with the manufacturer's color chart.

POLYMER COLOR SELECTION

Clear—   Clear deposits no color. It is designed to fill in the holes in the cuticle and create a smooth, flat surface that reflects light efficiently. This reflection of light gives the hair a shinier, healthier appearance.

Neutral—   Deposits a very low saturation of all three primary colors. Designed to create a smooth, flat surface that reflects light.

Red Base Color—   Deposits red tones that vary from copper to burgundy. Generally recommended for use on naturally brown and black hair.

Blue Base Color—   Deposits deep blue tones. Gives an iridescent blue glimmer to dark brown and black hair. On white hair, will look quite blue. Can turn green on yellow hair.

Green Base Color— Deposits ash tones. Good to neutralize excessive red. Not recommended for blonde or yellow hair.

Gold Base Color—   On blonde hair, deposits strong gold accents. On darker hair, leaves just a glint of gold.

Purple Base Color— On dark hair, leaves underlying plum tones. Can be diluted with clear to a pale violet for use as a neutralizer for excessive yellow in blonde hair.

Chemical Composition

Acetamide MEA, also known as n-acetyl acid amide or n-acetyl ethanolamine, is one of the main ingredients in many polymer colors. In crystal form, it works as a plasticizer, solvent, and stabilizer.

Propylene glycol, as used in cosmetics, is the most common moisture carrying vehicle other than water. It absorbs moisture and assists in the absorption of color. It dissolves oils and grease of the hair shaft for increased penetration. Propylene glycol is an inexpensive ingredient found in mascaras, spray deodorants, makeups, emollients, and suntan lotions.

Isostearamidopropyl dimethylamine lactate lowers water's surface tension, allowing the product to spread out and penetrate more easily. It is also commonly used in shampoos.

DMHF is the abbreviation for dimethyl hydantoin formaldehyde resin. Its purpose is to slowly liberate formaldehyde, which works as a preservative in the polymer colors. It is widely used as a germicide, fungicide, preservative, and embalming fluid.

Polyquaternium-10 is a member of the quaternary ammonium compound family. It is added to polymer colors for its abilities as a preservative, surfactant, and germicide. Diluted solutions are used in medicine as a sanitizer of skin and mucous membranes.

Cinnamyl alcohol is a crystalline alcohol made from cinnamon leaves and hyacinth oil. It serves as a pleasant scent in polymer colors as well as in many synthetic perfumes.

Benzophenone (1-12) has a delicate, rose-like fragrance and works to make the fragrance of the product last longer. It is a white flaky solid that is soluble in most oils. Also used in the manufacture of antihistamines and pesticides, benzophenone is toxic only if injected.

Thymol can be obtained from origanum, lavender, and a few other volatile oils. It is used in beauty aids, such as shampoos, toothpastes, mouthwashes, and polymer colors for its ability to destroy mold. Thymol also serves as a preservative for anatomical specimens and as a topical antifungal agent. It has a pleasant aroma, but is omitted from hypoallergenic cosmetics because it has a high incidence of allergic reaction.

Paraben derivatives are often used as preservatives in polymer colors. Methyl paraben is one of the most widely used preservatives in cosmetics as it inhibits the growth of a wide variety of microbes and is stable over the acid-alkaline range of most cosmetics. Propylparaben, or propyl p-hydroxybenzoate, is also used as a preservative and microbe inhibitor. Developed in Europe, propylparaben is used in shampoos, baby preparations, wave sets, eye lotions, hair-grooming aids, and medicinally to treat fungus.

Imidazolidinyl urea, a product of protein metabolism excreted from human urine, is probably, after the parabens, the most common preservative used in cosmetics. It effectively controls a wide range of germs in most pH bases. Odorless, tasteless, colorless, nontoxic, and nonirritating, imidazolidinyl urea is also used in eye shadows, permanent waves, fragrances, facial products, body lotions and oils, temporary rinses as well as polymer colors.

Xanthan is a gum produced by fermentation of a carbohydrate with a plant known as xanthomonas campestris. Xanthan is added to thicken polymer colors. This gum, also known as corn sugar gum, has no known toxicity.

Hydrolyzed protein is added to improve the condition of the hair after the color is removed. Hydrolyzing the protein, a chemical process in which the protein is made into a simpler compound, is done to increase its ability to stick to the natural protein of the hair.

Many of the colorants in polymer colors are FD&C approved; others are not. Direct, disperse, and certified dyes are found on the ingredient lists. The wide array of colors available to the colorist is made possible by the manufacturers' use of a great variety of these dyes. The exact formulation of these colors is considered a "trade secret" by the manufacturers, and therefore, by law, need not be divulged.

Safety

Polymer colors are compatible with other chemical services with the exception of bleaching to a very high stage. A highly saturated polymer can deposit such intense color that it is impossible to diffuse sufficiently with the products now available in the beauty industry, thus making correct toner development difficult if not impossible.

Most of the chemicals used in polymer colors are classified as safe by current research and regulation standards. However, a few of the ingredients, such as formaldehyde, may be considered suspect.

Researchers of the Division of Cancer Cause and Prevention of the National Cancer Institute indicated in April of 1983 that formaldehyde not only caused irritation to mucous membranes, but was also involved in DNA damage and reacted with other chemicals to cause mutation and cancer in cells. Its cosmetic use has been banned in Japan and Sweden, but very small amounts are still used in many American products even when it is *not* listed in the ingredients list.

Acetamide MEA is a mild skin irritant with low toxicity. However, it has caused liver cancer when ingested by rats in doses of 5000 milligrams per kilogram of body weight. Polyquaternium-10, like most quats, can be irritating if used in too strong a mixture and ingestion can be fatal.

The paraben derivatives, widely used as preservatives, can cause contact dermatitis. However, they are basically nonirritating, nonpoisonous, and non-sensitizing.

For the most part, polymer colors have at this point shown a low incidence of allergic reaction. Some manufacturers label their product as requiring a predisposition test; others do not. However, polymer colors do contain dyes that are not FDA approved, which does indicate a need for the allergy test.

POLYMER SEMIPERMANENT COLOR CHART

Objective

To create a chart of polymer colors that will serve as a ready reference for color selection.

Directions

Apply a polymer color on a small cotton ball. Work through and spread the cotton so that the color is apparent. Glue the cotton balls in the spaces indicated and write in the color name and the number in the space provided.

Brand used _____

#1 _____   #2 _____   #3 _____   #4_____

#5 _____   #6 _____   #7 _____   #8_____

9 _____   #10 _____   #11 _____   #12_____

#13 _____   #14 _____   #15 _____   #16_____

NATURAL POLYMER COLORS

EXPERIMENT INSTRUCTION SHEET

Objectives

To observe and document the color results of the natural polymer colors on virgin hair. To gain experience in color selection.

Hair Swatches Needed

- 4 virgin hair swatches—level 7 or 8
- 4 virgin hair swatches—level 4 or 5
- 4 virgin hair swatches—level 2 or 3

Labeling Hair Swatches

Label one swatch from each color group with the following:
- Clear
- Medium gold
- Soft brown
- Natural auburn

Materials Needed

- Polymer color products with the following bases: clear, medium gold, soft brown, and natural auburn
- Plastic bags

Procedure

1. Polymer colors are used just as they come out of the bottle. They require no additives or catalysts.
2. Thoroughly saturate one swatch of each color with one of the selected polymer colors.
3. Place the four swatches with the same polymer color on them in the same plastic bag and seal.
4. Process under a hot preheated dryer for 30 minutes.
5. Rinse thoroughly, until the water runs clear.
6. *If* manufacturer recommends, shampoo the hair.
7. Dry.
8. Mount swatches on the *Experiment Results Sheet on pages R-25 and R-27.*
9. Answer *Review Questions on page R-29.*

HIGH-FASHION POLYMER COLORS

EXPERIMENT INSTRUCTION SHEET

Objectives

To observe and document the color results of the high-fashion polymer colors on virgin hair. To gain experience in color selection.

Hair Swatches Needed

- 4 virgin hair swatches—level 7 or 8
- 4 virgin hair swatches—level 4 or 5
- 4 virgin hair swatches—level 2 or 3

Labeling Hair Swatches

Label one swatch from each color group with the following:
- Burgundy
- Deep red
- Blue
- Bright yellow

Materials Needed

- Polymer color products with the following bases: burgundy, deep red, blue, and bright yellow
- Plastic bags

Procedure

1. Polymer colors are used just as they come out of the bottle. They require no additives or catalysts.
2. Thoroughly saturate one swatch of each color with one of the selected polymer colors.
3. Place the four swatches saturated with the same polymer color in the same plastic bag and seal.
4. Process under a hot preheated dryer for 30 minutes.
5. Rinse thoroughly, until the water runs clear.
6. *If* manufacturer recommends, shampoo the hair.
7. Dry.
8. Mount swatches on the *Experiment Results Sheet on pages R-31 and R-33.*
9. Answer *Review Questions on page R-35.*

EFFECTS OF ARTIFICIAL HEAT ON POLYMER COLORS

EXPERIMENT INSTRUCTION SHEET

Objectives

To observe and document the difference in color results when the intensity and duration of heat varies in the processing of polymer colors.

Hair Swatches Needed

Two blonde and two brown swatches of hair in reasonably good condition

Labeling Hair Swatches

Label swatches accordingly:
- Light polymer color/low heat
- Light polymer color/high heat
- Dark polymer color/low heat
- Dark polymer color/high heat

Materials Needed

- Two polymer color products of your choice (one dark and one light)
- Plastic bags

Procedure

1. Polymer colors are used just as they come out of the bottle. They require no additives or catalysts.
2. Apply the light polymer color to the blonde swatches.
3. Apply the dark polymer color to the dark swatches.
4. Place each swatch in its own plastic bag and seal.
5. Process the one blonde and the one brown swatch in a preheated *warm* hood dryer for 10 minutes.
6. Process the other blonde and brown swatch in a preheated *hot* dryer for 30 minutes.
7. Rinse thoroughly, until the water runs clear.
8. *If* the manufacturer recommends, shampoo the hair.
9. Dry.
10. Mount swatches on the *Experiment Results Sheet on page R-37.*
11. Answer *Review Questions on page R-39.*

4

Permanent Hair Coloring Techniques

Permanent hair colors are prepared from a variety of materials: vegetables, flowers, herbs, salts of heavy metals, organic and synthetic chemicals. All of these permanent colors fall in one of the four classifications of permanent colors: vegetable tints, metallic dyes, compound dyestuffs, or oxidation tints.

VEGETABLE TINTS

In the past, before technology brought us the beauty industry as we now know it, many vegetable materials, such as lysimachia, logwood, indigo, chamomile, and henna were used as hair coloring ingredients.

Lysimachia

In ancient Rome, lysimachia was used to create a blonde tint. This plant, now known as the purple willow, was discovered by King Lysimachus of Thrace, a contemporary of Alexander the Great. It was highly prized by the predominantly dark haired Romans for its ability to lighten the hair.

Logwood

In the early 1900's, hairdressers would add a pinch of copper to set a dye, and then, for additional redness, another pinch of logwood. Logwood, or campeachy wood, is the product of the large and rapidly growing tree, Haematoxylon Campechianum, native to America, Cuba, Haiti, and the West Indies. Logwood is marketed in the form of a concentrated extract made from aged and fermented chips or raspings.

The coloring principle in logwood is haematoxylin. Haematoxylin is extracted by a chemical process that turns it to a large, transparent, sweet tasting crystal. When mixed with alkalies and metallic oxides, haematoxylin reacts to form other colors such as blues, greens, olives, and browns.

As well as a hair coloring, logwood is used to color fabrics. It has been particularly popular as a dye to create an inexpensive black colorant for cotton and wool fabrics and for its ability to render silk fiber opaque (a quality lacking in coal tar dyes).

Indigo

Indigo, the color of blue that is still popular today in the United States, is made from the leaves of a leguminous (from the pea family) plant. In the early days of its use, indigo was imported from India and Egypt. In 1649 it was planted in America with the hope that it would eventually become ten times more profitable than tobacco. While it never reached this goal, indigo has held a place of importance in the color industry with its use as a colorant for hair, inks, and textiles.

To make a dye, the leaves of the indigo plant are steeped for days in a mixture of fermenting fruit, wood ash, or urine. The resulting mixture is pale yellow and only when the dyed matter is aired does oxidation cause the color to appear.

Chamomile

Chamomile, or camomile, is an herb with hairy, slender, trailing, branched stems. The active ingredient used to make hair color is present in the flowering heads obtained from the Anethemis nobilis (Roman chamomile) or Matricaria chamomillae (German chamomile). The head of the flower is white with a yellow center, much like a daisy. Both the leaves and flowers of these plants have a strong though not unpleasant smell, but a very bitter and nauseous taste.

The active ingredient in the flowers of the chamomile is 1, 3, 4-trihydroxyflavone, also known as apigenin. Either an oily, aqueous extract or a paste of the ground flower heads may be used as a colorant.

When distilled from the flowers, the apigenin is also known as azulene for its deep blue color. This intensely blue hydrocarbon is still occasionally used in shampoo for both its color and fragrance. However, the less expensive, synthetic azulene now available is more commonly found on the ingredient list.

Chamomile flowers can be ground into a powder and used as a paste that is applied in a similar manner to a henna pack, with a processing time that ranges from 15-60 minutes. Used in this manner, it gives a lighter, brighter effect to the hair. Shampoos and rinses containing the powdered flowers are intended to add a bright yellow color in the hair. However, chamomile's effectiveness is disputed. A minimum concentration of 5 percent is necessary to produce any color change at all.

In the past, these powdered flowers have also been used as tonics and pain relievers. Extracts have been used as poultices to bring down swelling and inflammation, as well as highlighters for blonde hair. Currently, chamomile is used in cosmetics, skin fresheners, and ointments to soothe skin irritations.

Brewers sometimes use chamomile as a substitute for hops. The flowers have maintained a long history of popularity in the form of a tea that works as a diuretic and a medical treatment that increases perspiration. Ingestion of extremely large amounts may cause nausea and vomiting, but there is no known skin toxicity.

The chamomile in the United States was imported from Europe. Two close relatives of chamomile, May-weed or dog-fennel and corn chamomile, natives of Europe, have become naturalized American weeds.

Henna

The most noteworthy and popular of the vegetable colors comes from the plant known as Lawsonia alba, Lawsonia spinosa, and Lawsonia inermis, or more commonly, Egyptian privet or henna. Henna grows in moist climates throughout Africa, Arabia, Iran, and the East Indies.

Henna was first used by the inhabitants of those countries to dye their fingernails and the manes, hooves, and tails of their horses. For this purpose, leaves were removed before the flowering cycle, dried, ground into a fine powder, and hot water was added to create a paste. Application of this paste would impart a yellow color that needed refreshing every three to four weeks. Henna was also popular with the belly dancers who used it to color the palms of their hands and bottoms of their feet to accentuate the movements of their dance.

For use as a hair color, the ancient Egyptians blended henna powder with boiling water into a smooth, thin paste, and while still hot, brushed it onto the hair with a small stiff brush. Hot towels were then wrapped around the head and replaced as they cooled, for approximately half an hour. When the vegetable paste was removed with soap, brown hair was left with a bright chestnut color.

Henna is still used today to dye the red brown robes of the Masai tribesmen in Kenya, who proudly ignore the Western colors and styles even though, all around them, other tribes are giving into the influence. The use of henna has both ritual and cosmetic importance. Henna also is a functional part of current Moslem practice as it is used on hair, heads, and feet for its medicinal and strengthening powers as well as its beautifying abilities.

Henna is used by many dark-haired inhabitants of the tropics to provide relief from the heat. The addition of red tones to brown or black hair helps to reflect, rather than absorb, light rays.

Henna's uses are limited because of its narrow range of color possibilities. However, colorists have consistently experimented to expand its capabilities. In the early 1900's, hairdressers began adding logwood to create shades that were even redder than the natural hue of henna. To drab the red, they would rinse the hair with a solution of ¼ teaspoon of pyrogallic acid mixed in one quart of water. To darken the color, colorists would add just a pinch of Black Diamond Dye that was normally used for silk and wool. For the very darkest shades, they would add more acid and more dye. To lighten, a small amount of ammonia was added.

Henna and Gray Hair

Henna can be used on gray hair, but it generally is not recommended for hair that is more than 15 percent gray. The pure hennas will turn non-pigmented hair orange. The other shades of henna will all grab brighter than they would on pigmented hair.

Henna and Chemically Treated Hair

Henna is generally recommended for natural hair that has received no prior chemical treatments. However, a test strand will make the final determination whether or not a particular head can be successfully colored with henna. The more porous the hair shaft, the more drastic the color change will appear. Hair that has uneven porosity from scalp to ends may process unevenly with more color on the ends than at the scalp.

Bleached hair is too porous to accept henna properly. The henna powder is green. When applied to highly bleached hair, the color often remains green or at least reflects tinges of green. If the color does not process properly, the resulting color will be bright orange. Neutral or colorless henna is manufactured by a few companies for use on bleached hair.

Henna can interfere with permanent waving in two ways. First, the coating action of the color can build up to the point that the solution cannot penetrate properly. Second, henna penetrates and attaches to the salt bonds and leaves the bonds necessary for successful permanent waving unavailable for chemical alteration. The less often henna is used and the longer the time period between treatments, the more likely permanent waving will be successful.

The coating action of henna creates a hair strand that becomes thicker, and thus helps to give body to fine, limp hair. Because it makes no structural changes in the hair, it can be used on weak hair without damaging it. Henna fills in a roughened cuticle and holds together a split end to provide a slick, light-reflective surface. This, coupled with the addition of warmth, creates hair that shines. *(See Color Plates 21 and 22.)*

Although considered permanent, if used infrequently, the color will eventually shampoo out of the hair. This allows the client to experiment with auburn tones without committing to an oxidation tint.

Henna is a natural product that aesthetically appeals to the young client and the type of consumer that prefers organic products and avoids synthetics. Its "natural" qualities appeal to many.

However, it is important to remember that excessive application will build up on the outside of the shaft and can create an unnatural brassiness. If overused, the build-up can become so heavy that conditioners cannot penetrate to the hair shaft and the hair becomes dry and coarse.

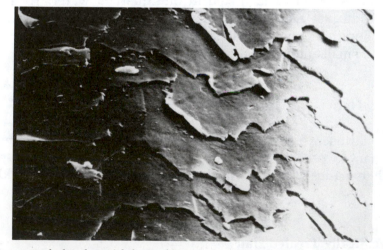

Henna attached to the cuticle layer of hair shaft.   (Courtesy: Redken Laboratories, Inc.)

Color Selection for Natural Hair

In selecting a color, the original hair color must be considered. Natural henna will add orange-red tones to the hair. Consult the manufacturer's literature for a particular brand's color selection.

Chemical and Physical Action of Henna

Henna penetrates into the cortical layer and also coats the cuticle of the hair shaft. A lasting color is created within the shaft when the pigment molecule of the henna combines with the S-bonds in the cortex. The coating action is small in the first application, but can increase to a build-up of color with repeated use.

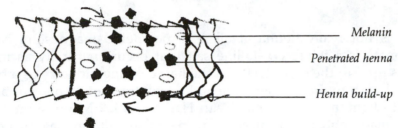

— *Melanin*
— *Penetrated henna*
— *Henna build-up*

Henna penetrates and coats the hair shaft.

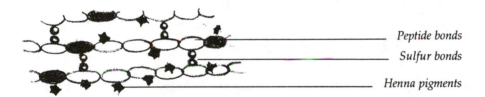

— *Peptide bonds*
— *Sulfur bonds*
— *Henna pigments*

Chemical Composition

Henna owes its hair dyeing abilities to the presence of 2-hydroxy-1,4-naphthaquinone, often termed *lawsone*. Lawsone is soluble in water and in an acid solution a substantial amount will adhere to the keratin of the hair shaft. Citric, adipic, or other acids are added to create the pH factor of 5.5 which is optimum for henna after it is mixed and ready for application.

Henna Reng

The addition of other substances to henna creates shades other than the natural auburn. The addition of indigo leaves to henna produces blue-black shades.

An aqueous formula for henna extract also utilizes the powdered flowers of the chamomile to deposit color. A typical formula is: powdered henna leaves, powdered chamomile flowers, pyrogallic acid, citric acid, alcohol, glycerin, and distilled water. The creation of this solution involves the infusion of henna powder, which extracts the active ingredient, lawsone. A substantial amount of this orange and red pigment will cling to keratin and has a coloring effect 100-150 times greater than that of powdered henna.

Today's Henna

Current technology has brought to the market hennas in black, chestnut, and auburn, plus a lightener. These hennas are made of concentrated herbal extracts titrated in tinctorial matters that have both a cumulative and a semipermanent effect. The dye coats the hair and is removed eventually by shampooing. The coloring is set by a complex between a natural alum and the flavenoids or the anthranaphtoquinones naturally present in plants. Under specific pH conditons, the complex is fixed onto keratinic fibers covering the external parts of the hair shaft. Application consists of a dispersion of the liquid hair dye into a gel made with *Amigel*, a natural polyglucose stable in the presence of salts and alcohol over the broad pH range of 2-12.

White Henna

White henna is not really henna at all. It is powdered magnesium carbonate. Magnesium carbonate is a white crystalline salt that occurs naturally as magnesite or dolomite. It was used in the early 1900's in the hair coloring industry as a bleaching agent. When mixed with hydrogen peroxide and a few drops of 28 percent ammonia, it could be used to lighten hair for that "Jean Harlow look." Magnesium carbonate can be artificially made and is also used in paint, table salt, and as an antacid. It does no harm on uninjured skin, but may cause irritation if applied over a cut or abrasion.

Safety

Henna enjoys a low incidence of skin irritation or allergic reaction, but should not be used over cuts or abrasions. It possesses no local or systemic toxicity. An occasional case of contact dermatitis is the only known adverse reaction to henna when applied to healthy, unbroken skin.

Henna is not always compatible with other chemical services. Read the manufacturer's recommended directions and perform a test strand before application to the entire head.

PURE HENNA

EXPERIMENT INSTRUCTION SHEET

Objectives

To observe and document the color resulting from pure vegetable henna application on natural hair.

Hair Swatches Needed

3 virgin hair swatches:

- Level 5 or 6
- Level 3 or 4
- Level 1 or 2

Labeling Hair Swatches

Label each swatch as to its natural color.

Materials Needed

- Pure vegetable henna
- Nonmetallic mixing receptacle
- Plastic wrap

Procedure

1. Place 1 tablespoon of henna in a nonmetallic mixing receptacle.
2. Add hot water to make a paste.
3. Apply henna to all three hair swatches.
4. Wrap in plastic wrap.
5. Process in a preheated dryer for 45 minutes.
6. Rinse, shampoo, and dry.
7. Mount swatches on the *Experiment Results Sheet on page R-41.*
8. Answer *Review Questions on page R-43.*

HENNA ADDITIVES

Just as in the early uses of henna, colorists still attempt to enhance and expand on the color selection available with hennas by the addition of other ingredients. The kitchen is a ready source of possibilities.

Mixing Synthetic Dyes with Henna

The standard training of a cosmetologist incorporates only a basic chemistry background. Therefore, it is recommended that no attempt be made to outguess the manufacturer's recommended mixing directions. Most manufacturers say to mix *nothing but natural organic ingredients* with henna whether the henna is natural or synthetic. Aniline derivative tints are definitely incompatible with henna. However, coloring with henna can be very creative with the addition of beet juice, cinnamon, paprika, and other items normally stocked in the pantry.

ORGANIC ADDITIVES FOR HENNA

Hair Color	Formula	Results
Light blonde	Neutral + ½ water replaced with lemon juice	Gold highlights
Medium and dark brown	Red henna + ½ water replaced with beet juice	Burgundy tones
Medium and dark brown	Red henna + 2 tbs. cinnamon	Cinnamon tones
Medium and dark brown	Red henna + ¼ vinegar + ¼ lemon juice + ½ water	Copper highlights
Medium and dark brown	Red henna + 2 tbs. allspice	Richer brown
Medium and dark brown	Red henna + 2 tbs. nutmeg	Richer brown
Medium and dark brown	Red henna + 2 tbs. paprika	Redder peppery color

---

PURE HENNA WITH ORGANIC ADDITIVES

EXPERIMENT INSTRUCTION SHEET

Objectives

To observe and document the color changes occurring from the mixing of organic additives to pure henna.

Hair Swatches Needed

Six swatches of level 2, 3, or 4 that have received no prior color treatments.

Labeling Hair Swatches

Swatches will be labeled according to the organic additive included in the formula used on it.

- Beet juice
- Cinnamon

- Vinegar and lemon juice
- Allspice
- Nutmeg
- Paprika

Materials Needed

- 2 teaspoons beet juice
- 1 teaspoon vinegar
- Nutmeg
- Cinnamon
- 1 teaspoon lemon
- Allspice
- Paprika
- Pure natural henna
- Plastic wrap
- Nonmetallic mixing receptacles

Product Formulation

1. *Formula #1*—Place 2 teaspoons beet juice and 2 teaspoons hot water in nonmetallic mixing receptacle. Add henna to make a paste.
2. *Formula #2*—Place 1 teaspoon vinegar, 1 teaspoon lemon juice, and 2 teaspoons hot water in a nonmetallic mixing receptacle. Add henna to make a paste.
3. *Formula #3*—Mix 1 teaspoon of henna and a sprinkle of allspice in a nonmetallic mixing receptacle. Add hot water to make a paste.
4. *Formula #4*—Mix 1 teaspoon of henna and a sprinkle of cinnamon in a nonmetallic mixing receptacle. Add hot water to make a paste.
5. *Formula #5*—Mix 1 teaspoon of henna and a sprinkle of nutmeg in a nonmetallic mixing receptacle. Add hot water to make a paste.
6. *Formula #6*—Mix 1 teaspoon of henna and a sprinkle of paprika in a nonmetallic mixing receptacle. Add hot water to make a paste.

Procedure

1. Apply a different formulation to each swatch as indicated on the label.
2. Wrap each swatch separately in plastic wrap.
3. Process in a preheated dryer for 45 minutes.
4. Rinse, shampoo, and dry.
5. Mount swatches on the *Experiment Results Sheet on page R-45.*
6. Answer *Review Questions on page R-47.*

REMOVAL OF HENNA BUILD-UP

Sometimes it is possible to remove henna when it becomes excessively built up on the shaft or when it is incompatible with a future chemical service. The following procedure outlines the steps to remove henna build-up.

Application Procedure

1. Apply 70 percent alcohol to the hair shaft, avoiding direct contact with the scalp. Allow to set 5-7 minutes.
2. Apply mineral oil directly over the alcohol, completely saturating each strand from scalp to ends.
3. Preheat hood dryer.
4. Tightly cover the head with a plastic bag.
5. Place under dryer for 30 minutes.
6. Without rinsing, apply concentrated shampoo for oily hair and work into the oil.
7. Allow to set in hair for 3 minutes.
8. Massage hair again.
9. Add comfortably hot water and rinse thoroughly.
10. Shampoo again. (Three shampoos may be necessary.)

Technically the alcohol should loosen the henna coating the hair shaft. However, more than one treatment may be necessary to loosen it enough to slide off. Always perform a test strand to determine if removal was successful before applying the next chemical treatment.

Removal of Henna from Facial Hair

The lighter, more porous facial hairs can easily grab too much color. To loosen some of the excess, saturate the hair with 70 percent alcohol and process 3 minutes. Then follow with a mineral oil. Let set another 3 minutes and apply a concentrated shampoo for oily hair. Rinse and shampoo until oil is completely removed. Apply a second time if color removal is insufficient, but only apply in the areas of excess color coating.

Removal of Henna Odor

Henna has an earthy, herbal odor that often lingers in the hair after shampooing. To eliminate this odor, use an acid-balanced (approximately 5.0-6.0) shampoo for the final sudsing. If odor still remains, rinse the hair with a cider-vinegar rinse. If this is still unsuccessful, try a tomato juice rinse.

METALLIC HAIR DYES

Metallic hair colors can be recognized by the descriptive terms used by manufacturers in their packaging even before reading the ingredients list. Metallic dyes are known as "progressive hair colors" and "color restorers." They are referred to as progressive because the hair progressively turns darker and darker upon each subsequent application. The term color restorer is used because the "natural" color of the hair *appears* to be gradually restored.

History

Metallic salts were a common ingredient in hair color formulations prior to the 1900's. However, their use was highly curtailed as evidence accumulated indicating that structural and chemical damage, leading to hair breakage and loss, resulted from extended periods of use of these products.

Many episodes of physical illness were attributed by physicians of the time to the use of metallic hair colors. Nausea, headaches, and even lead poisoning seemed to be related to extensive use of hair colors with a high concentration of metallic salts.

Metallic hair dyes comprise a minor portion of the home hair coloring market and currently are never used professionally. Nevertheless, it is crucial for the professional colorist to be informed of the chemical composition, characteristics, and methods of removal because metals react adversely with oxidation solutions.

Clients occasionally request chemical services without knowing the incompatibility of metallic color with professional products. Consumers generally do not even realize that they used a product containing metal. The colorist must be able to analyze and prescribe safe, professional treatments to avoid hair damage and discoloration.

Color Selection

Metallic hair dyes offer no color selection. The exact shade achieved depends upon the concentration of metallic salts in the solution, the number of applications, the original color of the hair, and the processing time.

Metallic dyes are intended for daily application over a week or so in a manner that creates a gradual color change. The shades produced in gray hair usually pass through many levels from yellow to brown or black. When the desired color is reached, the consumer is to reduce the frequency of application to maintain the color. While these products are intended to be used frequently, such use tends to dull the hair, creating flat, unnatural-looking shades.

Chemical and Physical Action

The colors produced by metallic salts are due to sulfides formed by the reaction between the sulfur in the keratin and the metallic salts and to metallic oxides formed by the keratin reducing the metal salts. The metallic salts react with the sulfur of the hair keratin, eventually turning the protein brown. In this reaction, the quality of the keratin is lowered from the use of this chemical.

The physical result is a colored film coating the hair shaft, which gives the hair a characteristic dull metallic appearance. The metallic coating also builds up on the surface of the hair shaft and creates a darker and darker appearance with each subsequent use. Repeated treatments leave the hair brittle and conflict with future chemical services that include in their formulation urea peroxide, hydrogen peroxide, sodium perborate, thioglycolate, ammonia and/or most other oxidizers.

Chemical Composition

Metallic dyes are chemically classified as "pre-metallized dyes." These dyes are currently used more commonly on fabrics than hair.

The active ingredient in lead dyes is usually lead acetate in a solution including

sulfur, glycerin, and water. A typical, yet unstable, formula is:
- Rose-water—87.5 percent
- Glycerin—6 to 9 percent
- Lead acetate—1 to 6 percent
- Sulfur—1 to 3 percent

Lead acetate, also known as sugar of lead, is a white crystal with a sharp, sour odor. It has also been used to treat bruises and skin irritations in animals. While lead acetate is the most common metallic salt used, a few colorants in solutions with bismuth, silver, copper, nickel, and cobalt do presently exist.

In addition to their use in hair colorings, bismuth compounds, subgallate, subnitrate, and oxychloride, may be found on the ingredient list of a variety of cosmetics such as bleaching and freckle creams, skin protectants, antiseptics, dusting powders, eye shadows and blushes, or any "frosted" products. Bismuth compounds are odorless and tasteless.

Bismuth citrate is an approved color additive, but is used to a much lesser extent than lead acetate. It is a gray-white powder with a bright metallic luster occurring naturally in the earth's crust. In the past bismuth citrate was used to treat syphilis.

Silver is a white metal used in hair coloring for its germicidal effects as well as its ability to speed up the process without changing itself. Prolonged absorption of silver compounds will cause a grayish-blue discoloration on the skin and hair.

Silver nitrate and silver sulfate both act as germicides, antiseptics, and astringents in cosmetics as well as serving as coloring agents in metallic hair dyes. The white crystalline salts of silver were especially popular for use in the production of nineteenth-century dyes. Silver colors the hair by combining with keratin. The exposure to light and organic matter at the same time causes it to darken and turn brown.

Copper, in the form of a metallic powder, is also known as versenate. It is used as a coloring agent in many cosmetics besides metallic dyes. Copper is an essential nutrient for all mammals. Copper deficiency leads to anemia, skeletal defects, and muscle degeneration.

Nickel sulfate is used in astringents and nickel plating as well as metallic hair colorings. It is found naturally in the earth's crust as a salt of nickel in green or blue crystals. Nickel sulfate has a sweet astringent taste that is deceptive of its true nature.

Safety

The Federal Food and Drug Administration reports that complaints against metallic hair dyes include headaches, scalp irritation, contact dermatitis, facial swelling, hair breakage and loss, lead poisoning, and explosion of the bottles of dye.

Lead dyes are used in the formulation of progressive hair dyes through permission given by the FDA even though these dyes are proven carcinogens (capable of causing cancer). Lead has the ability to be absorbed through the skin, build up within the system, and thus lead to either cancer or lead poisoning.

Nickel is a common cause of skin rashes. It can be extremely toxic and cause vomiting if swallowed. Its systemic effects include nervous depression, brain, kidney, and blood vessel damage.

Silver compounds are highly poisonous. Copper salts, especially copper sulfates, are highly irritating to skin and mucous membranes. Ingestion causes violent vomiting.

Metallic dyes are not compatible with most oxidizers, and therefore are not compatible with most other chemical services. All these metallic salts cause a dramatic increase of the kinetic molecular movement within the hair shaft, which creates a rise in temperature of the products upon application of an oxidizing agent. Resulting damage has been discoloration, breakage, poor permanent waving results, and even destruction to the point of a melted hair shaft due to the heat created in this adverse chemical reaction.

This type of color, sold for home use, poses a health risk when any of the metallic salts, but lead in particular, remains on the hands and is ingested through oral contact or through the contamination of food. Ingestion, especially by children, could prove fatal. Therefore, this product should be stored well out of the reach of small children.

TESTING FOR METALLIC DEPOSITS ON THE HAIR SHAFT

EXPERIMENT INSTRUCTION SHEET

Objectives

To determine what the exact chemical and physical reaction will be on hair, if the colorist suspects that metallic coloring was used, before applying further chemical treatments.

Hair Swatches Needed

- Several swatches treated with a variety of metallic colors
- 1 virgin hair swatch
- If you separate each of the swatches treated with metallic colors into two parts and save half, you will be prepared for the next experiment, *Removal of Metallic Dyes on page 72.*

Materials Needed

- 1 ounce 20 volume H_2O_2
- 20 drops of 28 percent ammonia water
- Nonmetallic mixing receptacle

Procedure

1. Add 1 ounce of 20 volume hydrogen peroxide to 20 drops of 28 percent ammonia water in a nonmetallic mixing receptacle.
2. Dunk hair swatch in solution. Allow to process in the solution for 30 minutes.
3. Remove swatch from solution and allow to set for 24 hours.
4. Mount swatches on the *Experiment Results Sheet on page R-49.*

Reading Test Results

1. *Virgin Hair* will lighten *slightly* after 30 minutes in the solution, but there will be no breakage or undue damage at the end of the 24 hours.

2. *Lead Deposits* are indicated by an immediate lightening of the hair swatch. The strand will not appear excessively weakened or suffer any breakage.
3. *Silver Deposits* are indicated by a lack of change because the solution cannot penetrate the coating.
4. *Copper Deposits* are indicated by a disagreeable rotten egg-like smell. Both the solution and the hair strand will become very hot within moments of saturation. The strand will seem to almost "melt" because it becomes so weak that it will break when pulled at the end of 24 hours, if not sooner.

REMOVAL OF METALLIC DYES

EXPERIMENT INSTRUCTION SHEET

Objectives

An attempt may be made to remove metallic dyes from the hair shaft, but these attempts may or may not be effective. Performing a test strand will indicate whether or not the metallic deposits have been removed. If not, the entire application must be repeated until the hair shaft is sufficiently free of metal salts to perform other chemical services.

Hair Swatches Needed

- Several swatches treated with metallic dyes. (The swatches you saved and did *not* use to test for metallic deposits in the previous experiment may be reused for this test.)

Materials Needed

- 70 percent alcohol
- Concentrated shampoo for oily hair
- Mineral, castor, vegetable, or commercially prepared color removing oil

Procedure

1. Apply 70 percent alcohol to each dry hair swatch with a cotton ball.
2. Allow alcohol to stand for 5 minutes.
3. Apply the heavy oil thoroughly to the hair swatches.
4. Cover hair completely with plastic bag.
5. Place swatches under hot dryer for 30 minutes.
6. To remove, saturate swatches with concentrated shampoo.
7. Work shampoo into oil for 3 minutes, then rinse with warm water.
8. Repeat shampoo steps until oil is completely removed.
9. Mount these swatches next to the swatches that were tested for metallic deposits on the *Experiment Results Sheet on page R-49*, noting that these swatches are assumed to be free of metallic dyes.
10. Answer *Review Questions on page R-51.*

COMPOUND DYESTUFF

Compound dyestuff is a combination of vegetable and metallic dyes. Metallic salts are added to the vegetable dyes as a fixative to increase color fastness, thus creating a formulation that has more staying power. In addition, the metallic salts create new and different colors than those available with pure vegetable tints.

The most common example of a compound dye is compound henna. Some compound hennas on the market today still utilize the same basic formula created hundreds of years ago. A typical formula is a mixture of powdered henna, pyrogallic acid, and copper sulfate. Compound dyes are no longer used in the professional cosmetology industry. However, they are still available to the consumer at many drug, grocery, and discount stores.

Vegetable dyes have the tendency to look unnatural because they build up on the outside of the hair shaft. This build-up interferes with the normal reflection of light and gives the hair a flat, dull appearance. The metallic salts cause the vegetable tint to adhere and build up even more. In addition, metallic salts can cause discoloration and brittleness to the hair. When the metallic deposits are excessive, breakage and destruction of the hair shaft may occur.

Before any chemical application, if the colorist suspects that a compound dye has been used, the *Test for Metallic Salts* should be given on a hair sample. If the test proves positive, the metallic salts should be removed with the procedure outlined for use on a hair swatch under *Removal of Metallic Salts on page 72.*

OXIDATION TINTS

Oxidation tints have been available since 1883. Originally designed to color animal furs, which are a type of hard keratin similar in structure to human hair, oxidation tints were first used as a hair coloring in 1885 but did not become widely used and socially acceptable until the 1950's.

Permanent hair dyes, on a professional level, are based almost entirely on the use of oxidation tints. Commercially these dyes are known by a variety of names: para-dyes, aniline derivative tints, permanent tints, synthetic-organic tints, penetrating tints, amino tints, cream tints, and tube colors, as well as oxidation tints.

The term "para-dye" refers to the colorless substances, either paraphenylenediamine or paratoluenediamine, that transform into a colored material in and on the hair shaft as a consequence of the chemical reactions that occur when mixed with an oxidizer such as hydrogen peroxide. Even though some oxidation tints no longer contain either of these derivatives, "para-dye" has become a term that refers to all oxidation tints regardless of chemical composition.

"Aniline derivative tint" refers to the fact that aniline is a derivative of coal tar. "Synthetic-organic" indicates that aniline is a compound synthetically conceived (man-made) from an organic (found naturally in nature) compound.

"Penetrating tint" is a term descriptive of the ability of a tint after it is mixed with its oxidizer to penetrate through the cuticle and into the cortex layer of the hair shaft. "Amino" refers to the protein chain which can be included in the formulation of a tint, while "cream" refers to the consistency of the product. "Tube color" is a term that describes the packaging of the coloring product.

Permanent hair color can be formulated and packaged in either solution, emulsion, gel, shampoo, powder, tablet, or even stick form. This form is known as the vehicle. The main purpose of the vehicle is to distribute the dye mixture evenly throughout the hair. Technology has brought the color industry to the point that nearly any shade can be created on hair utilizing the variety of available dye intermediates, modifiers, and oxidizing agents.

Oxidation dyes can lighten and deposit color in one application, a feat performed by no other color classification. This ability to create an infinite array of hues, levels, and saturations has made permanent colors irreplaceable in the industry.

Tint Versus Dye

The literal definition of tint is "a delicate color or hue; a tinge; a color with reference to its mixture with white." However, the word "tint" has been adapted, mainly for advertising purposes, by the cosmetology industry to mean the same as "dye."

"Dye" is defined as a product or substance used to color fabric, hair, etc. The word "dye" is not readily accepted by consumers. It retains its association with the metallic and vegetable dyes used in the past, which produced unnatural looking hair color that left the hair dry and damaged. The consumer also relates the term "dye" to the method used to color clothing and does not like to know that some of the same chemicals and processes used in fabric dyes are also used to color the hair.

The word "dyeing" has also been subliminally confused with "dying." This can lead consumers to the assumption that dyeing does irreparable harm to the hair and can "kill" a sale! Therefore, the word "tint," with its pleasant connotations, is a more successful sales tool.

Chemical and Physical Reaction

In a permanent dye, the chemical ingredients that create the physical reaction within the hair shaft are divided into three categories: *bases* or *primary intermediates, couplers* or *modifiers,* and *oxidizers.*

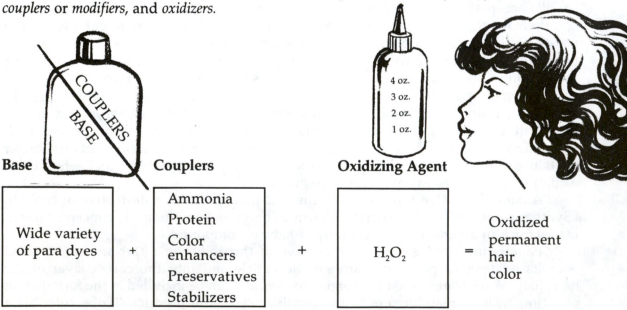

Base		Couplers		Oxidizing Agent	
Wide variety of para dyes	+	Ammonia Protein Color enhancers Preservatives Stabilizers	+	H_2O_2	= Oxidized permanent hair color

Bases or Primary Intermediates are synthetic organic chemicals, which in a chemical action with the couplers and oxidizing agent create artificial pigment. All oxidation dyes are based on synthetic organic chemicals or dye intermediates. Paraphenylenediamine and paratoluenediamine are used more often than other available dye intermediates, either singly or in various blends to produce a wide range of shades.

Couplers or Modifiers are the ingredients added to obtain certain colors, to improve the stability of the dye, to improve the finished condition of the hair shaft, and to preserve the product.

Oxidizing Agents can be urea peroxide or melamine peroxide. However, hydrogen peroxide is the most popular.

Both paraphenylenediamine and paratoluenediamine can be analyzed to find that they describe the exact nature of each molecule. "Para" is a prefix meaning "opposite" such as in parallel and paradox. "Di" is a prefix meaning "twice" such as in dioxide and dimension. This means that both have a tint-base molecule (phenylene or toluene) that has two (di) free arms (amine) that are opposite (para) each other.

The commercially packaged dye or tint contains the bases and the couplers. The colorist adds the oxidizing agent to create a chemical reaction. This reaction, which occurs at the alkaline pH created to a great extent by the ammonia in the packaged dye solution, is known as oxidation. This oxidizer chemically joins together the aimine groups or free arms of adjacent molecules.

Application of this oxidizing tint in an alkaline state causes the hair shaft to swell and the cuticle to open. The molecules of the tint base, before mixing with the oxidizer, are very small. These small colorless bases or intermediates can pass easily through the cuticle and into the cortex of the hair shaft. As the oxidation process begins, the coupling together of hundreds of the small colorless tint-base molecules changes them into large chains of colored, relatively stable pigment.

These molecules become trapped beneath the cuticle as they are now too large to be shampooed out. Furthermore, they form acid bonds with the keratin chains in the cortex and become part of the hair structure. This formation of acid bonds, rather than affixing to the H-bonds and S-bonds, creates permanent color while leaving the hair with the ability to be permanently waved or relaxed with certain care and precaution. The end product of this oxidation process is an azine dye that reacts with the keratin of the hair shaft to form insoluble azine derivatives that become permanent color. *(See Color Plates 23 and 24.)*

Chemical Composition of the Bases or Primary Intermediates

The bases of oxidation tints are aromatic (fragrant) compounds, almost exclusively benzene derivatives. Benzene is a solvent obtained from coal. It is also used in nail polish removers, varnishes, lacquers, and as a solvent for waxes, resins, and oils. The most commonly used compounds from this classification are:

- *p-phenylenediamine*
- *o-phenylenediamine*
- *p-aminophenol*
- *o-aminophenol*
- *p-dihydroxybenzene*
- *o-dihydroxybenzene*

- *p-toluenediamine (2,5-toluenediamine, p-toluylenediamine or p-tolylenediamine)*
- *p-aminodiphenylamine*
- *p-diaminoanisole*

Chemical Composition of the Couplers or Modifiers

Many permanent hair dyes include ammonia in the formulation to activate the coloring process. Ammonia is obtained by blowing steam through incandescent coke. It is also used in permanent waves, bleaches, and in the manufacture of fabrics and explosives.

Ammonia, as formulated into oxidation tints, has the disadvantages of a strong odor and the ability to aggressively attack melanin, often causing excessive color diffusion and structural damage.

The industry has taken strides to manufacture tint products that either replace or partially replace ammonia. However, the permanent tints containing no ammonia do not have the lifting power of those formulated with it.

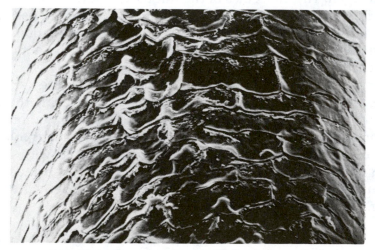

High-lift tint damage.   *(Courtesy Redken Laboratories, Inc.)*

One manufacturer replaces ammonia with peptides rich in arginine or guanidine. Although strongly alkaline, both are less aggressive to the hair shaft than ammonia. Arginine is an essential amino acid that plays an important part in the production of urea excretion. It is also currently used for the treatment of liver diseases. Guanidine is a colorless crystal that dissolves in water. It is found in earthworms, mussels, rice hulls, mushrooms, and turnip juice. Guanidine is a muscle poison if ingested but is not toxic on the surface of the skin.

Morpholine is also a peptide used to replace ammonia. It is made by taking the water out of the alcohol known as diethanolamine. Morpholine has a strong ammonia odor but is not as damaging to the hair structure as ammonia. It has also been used as an emulsifier in cosmetics, a corrosion inhibitor, an insecticide, a local anesthetic, and an antiseptic.

A variety of alkanolamines are also available to replace ammonia. These are compounds comprised of alcohols from alkene (a saturated fatty hydrocarbon) and amines (from ammonia). Alkanolamines are also used in cold creams, eyeliners, and soaps. They have no known toxicity.

Triethanolamine and diethylamine can also be used to create an alkaline state. The principal toxic effect of triethanolamine in tests on animals is due to its over-alkalinity. It is also used as a coating agent for fresh fruit and vegetables, as well as being widely used as a surfactant. Diethylamine is prepared from methanol and ammonia. It is very soluble in water and, like triethanolamine, forms a strong alkali. Diethylamine is also used in detergent soaps and has proven to be irritating to the skin and mucous membranes.

Benzene serves as a primary ingredient of the bases of oxidation tints. 1,3-benzene is a solvent obtained from coal that is also used in the manufacture of varnish, nail polish remover, lacquer, detergents, nylon, artificial leather, antiknock agents in gasoline, airplane fuel, and as a solvent for waxes and resins.

The anti-oxidant protects the dye system from oxidation due to contact with the atmosphere during manufacture and packaging. It also slows down the oxidation process during the preparatory time of mixing the hydrogen peroxide into the formula. Sodium sulfite or thioglycolic acid can be used as anti-oxidants.

Sodium sulfite is a white to tannish pink salt found in crystal and powder form. It has a salty sulfur-like taste. As well as serving as an anti-oxidant in hair dyes and bleaches, it is used as an antiseptic, preservative, and a topical anti-fungus medicine. Sodium sulfite can be drying, but has no known skin toxicity.

Thioglycolic acid is better known for its work in areas other than hair coloring, such as its use in permanent waves and relaxers. Thioglycolic acid is made by a complex chemical reaction of two sodium compounds. A solution of .1-1.0 percent is used as an alternative to sodium sulfite, particularly in cream preparations. Ammonium thioglycolic acid stabilizes the dye and has a reducing effect upon keratin. This effect has led to preparations and techniques that combine a dyeing process with permanent waving. However, thio must be handled carefully as it can cause hair breakage, pustules, irritations, and allergic reactions.

A variety of enzymes also effectively inhibit premature oxidation of para dye bases. An enzyme is an organic substance, such as ascorbic acid, produced in plant and animal cells that causes changes in other substances by catalytic action.

Ascorbic acid (vitamin C) is best known for its controversial abilities to prevent and cure the common cold. It is reasonably stable but deteriorates rapidly when exposed to air while mixed in an aqueous solution. Therefore, it probably is not as effective as an anti-oxidant as some of the other chemicals used for this purpose.

Ammonium carbonate, different than ammonia, is a salt that is found in nature. It is an odorless crystal or powder that has a salty taste. Ammonium carbonate is used as an acidifier in many tints and permanent waves as well as in the manufacture of batteries, explosives, and medicines.

Oleic acid is a colorless oil that assists with pH adjustment and penetration of the product. It is obtained from animal and vegetable fats and oils. It is commonly used in the cosmetic industry in makeup, liquid lip color, and shampoo.

Ceteth, or polyethylene cetyl ether, is a compound of a variety of derivatives of alcohols. It is used as a component of the detergent found in oxidation tints. It also inhibits the growth of fungus in the product.

A variety of the glycols, as well as plain glycol, are regular additives to oxidation tint formulas. Glycol literally means "glycerine plus alcohol." It is a group of syrupy alcohols that are widely used in cosmetics as humectants. The various glycols have additional unique characteristics as described below.

Propylene glycol, commercially known as 1,2-propanediol, is also added to increase the penetration of a product. It is the most common moisture-carrying ingredient used in cosmetics other than water itself. It absorbs moisture and acts as a solvent and wetting agent. Propylene glycol is used in a wide variety of cosmetics, foundations, mascaras, cold creams, lipsticks, perfumes, suntan lotions, shaving lotions, and hair straighteners.

The use of butylene glycol has the advantage of preserving against spoilage. It is made from acetylene formaldehyde and hydrogen. Even though all formaldehyde products are suspect, as used in cosmetics, butylene glycol exhibits no toxicity.

Polyethylene glycol (PEG) works as a solvent, softener, binder, and plasticizing agent in pharmaceutical ointments as well as the cosmetic items listed for propylene glycol. It improves resistance to moisture and oxidation. PEG is combustible, but nontoxic to man.

Ethoxydiglycol is also used for its solvent abilities. It is a liquid prepared from petroleum, and like most petroleum products, has a fairly high incidence of allergic reaction.

Distilled water is occasionally added to oxidation tints to act as a solvent. However, it is rarely used alone because the dye intermediates have a low solubility in water.

Another improvement in the formulation of oxidation tints has been the increase in the light stability of the toluenediamine-recorcinol preparation by the addition of diamino-1,2 (manufactured from aniline) or 1,3-benzene (obtained from coal tar) as well as the addition of an ultra violet filter such as benzylidine-camphor or dodecyl benzotriazoles. These ingredients give hair coloring a longer shelf life as they are less affected by natural and artificial light.

To achieve permanent dyeing of the hair shaft it is necessary to inflict some structural damage. To inhibit this damage or to restore the original condition of the hair, the following substances are commonly included in the formulation of oxidation tints: keratin hydrolysates (keratose obtained by hot treatment of keratin materials with aqueous bases), methylol derivatives (from an alkyl imidazolone associated with amidobetaine), or Miranol (polyesters of polycarboxylic cycloaliphatic or aromatic acids of polyalkylene oxides).

Some lines of hair coloring utilize the quaternary ammonium compounds for the purpose of improving the aesthetic qualities of the hair after coloring. The quaternary ammonium compounds leave the hair easy to comb and improve its general appearance. The QUATS are widely used in most areas of cosmetic manufacture as preservatives, surfactants, germicides, antiseptics, deodorants, and sanitizers. They can be toxic in strong solutions and have been known to irritate the skin. Tallowamidopropyl chloride, or tallow trimethyl ammonium chloride, and benzyltrimonium chloride are two of the QUATS most commonly used in oxidation tints.

PVP, or polyvinlypyrrolidone, is a solid plastic resin that is also used in shampoos, hair sprays, and lacquers. It closely resembles the structure and action of a group of simple proteins that is usually derived from egg white. When the water evaporates from the mixture, the PVP gives a tight, slick feeling to the surface of the hair shaft. The use of PVP in hair sprays has been controversial because it is believed to produce lung problems when inhaled. Both ingestion and injection of PVP have been proven to cause health problems. However, due to the method of application used, neither of these is likely in hair coloring services.

In addition to PVP, a whole series of vinyl polymers falling under the general classification of methacrylates and acrylates are used by some manufacturers to improve the outward condition of the hair. These polymers, such as vinyl acetate and vinyl chloride, are made from the reaction between acetylene and certain compounds such as alcohol, phenol, and amines. They create a surface coating on the hair shaft and are used for the same purpose in false nails, nail lacquer preparations, plastics, and synthetic fibers.

Amodimethicone is a silicone polymer containing amino acids. It coats and protects the hair shaft from moisture. In addition to its use in tints, amodimethicone is also used in waterproofing and lubrications as well as in beauty products such as nail driers, hand lotions, protective creams, and hair straighteners.

Acrylamide is a colorless, odorless crystal that is also added to hair color to improve the manageability of the hair after the treatment. As well, it is used in the manufacture of adhesives, nail polishes, face masks, and permanent-press fabrics.

Isopropyl alcohol, or isopropanol, is an antibacterial agent and a solvent used to dissolve oils for better penetration of the product. Isopropyl alcohol is denatured meaning that it was purposely given a terrible taste to discourage ingestion. However, other ingredients in tint already make the product extremely unappetizing, so it is rarely added for this purpose.

Methylisothiazolinone is used in conjuction with methylchloroisothiazolinone as a preservative in oxidation tints as a replacement for formaldehyde. While formaldehyde has well-known toxicity, little is known about either of these new additives.

Resorcinol works in conjunction with paraphenylenediame to create color within the cortex. It doubles as a preservative, anti-fungus, antiseptic, astringent, and anti-itch ingredient. Resorcinol has a sweet taste.

Naphthas is a coupler that also creates color when combined with paraphenyl-enediame. 1-Naphthol and 2-naphthol are two common products of naphthas sometimes found on tint ingredient lists. 2-Naphthol is important because of its ability to darken gray hair.

A wide variety of the aminophenols are used in brown oxidation tints. Aminophenol is a colorless crystal derived from phenol (carbolic acid), which is made from coal tar. While this compound can cause a lack of oxygen in the blood, it is considered less toxic than aniline.

Octoxynol, or polyoxyethylene octylphenyl ether, is added to increase the detergent content of the product and as an emulsifier and dispersing agent. It is also used in lipsticks and hand creams. Octoxynol has no known toxicity.

Nonoxynol is also used as a dispersing agent and doubles as an emulsifying surface-active agent. It has no known toxicity.

Coleth=24 is also added to oxidation tints as an emulsifier. It is a derivative of cholesterol that has no known toxicity.

Linoleamide DEA is a derivative of linoleic acid, which is an essential fatty acid prepared from edible fats and oils. Like the two ingredients above, it works as an emulsifier, but also has emollient properties. It is a common ingredient in vitamins, especially vitamin F. Large doses can cause nausea, but it has no known skin toxicity.

Sodium lauryl sulfate is a detergent or surfactant found on many shampoo ingredient listings and also commonly found in shampoo based oxidation tints. It assists in easy removal of the product. The degreasing abilities of sodium lauryl sulfate may cause dryness to the skin and hair, but it is generally nonallergenic and nontoxic.

Triethanolamine also serves as a surfactant. It is very alkaline and is toxic if taken internally in substantial doses. Unbelievable as it may seem, triethanolamine is used by the food industry as a coating agent for fresh fruit and vegetables.

Cocamidopropylamine oxide is a derivative of coconut oil, taken from the white, semisolid, highly saturated fat kernels of the coconut. It aids in the lathering qualities of the product and works as a cleanser.

Sulfonated or sulfated castor oil works to keep the mixture together and as a wetting agent in oxidation tints as well as soapless shampoos and hair sprays. It attracts other oils and may dry the skin and hair.

Combination of the Base and Coupler

The colors created by oxidation dyes are a result of the combination of a variety of bases and couplers. Infinite possibilities exist for the creation of new hues as more than one (often a dozen or more) base and coupler combinations are used in each formula. The list below gives examples of the colors created by the combination of p-phenylenediamine with a variety of couplers:

COUPLER	*COLOR OBTAINED*
Resorcinol	Green/brown
m-aminophenol	Magenta/brown
2,4,diaminoanisole and m-phenylenediamine	Blue
1-naphthol	Purple/blue

Chemical Composition of the Oxidizer

While other oxidizers are available, hydrogen peroxide is the oxidizing agent used almost exclusively with today's permanent tints. It is generally chosen by most manufacturers over melamine peroxide and urea peroxide because hydrogen peroxide is efficient when combined with the bases and couplers, but also for its ability to promote the simultaneous decolorization of the hair being tinted.

This lightening occurs simultaneously with, but independent of, the dyeing. It results in the natural pigment being lightened sufficiently to allow the desired color development of the artificial tint. The degree of lightening depends on the ratio of hydrogen peroxide added to the alkali, such as ammonia, contained in the packaged dye. For example, a dye intended to lighten one level will contain approximately 15 percent ammonia to 20 percent hydrogen peroxide. A solution of 15 percent ammonia mixed with a 30 volume hydrogen peroxide will give a higher lift to the natural pigment. In some cases, the amount of hydrogen peroxide and ammonia is more than necessary for the oxidation process. This causes excessive damage to the cuticle and cortex, and over diffuses the melanin within the shaft.

Hydrogen peroxide is one of the most important components of the hair coloring industry. It is used in conjunction with many products. The history, theory, and chemistry of this ingredient is covered in the Chapter titled "Hydrogen Peroxide."

Safety of Oxidation Tints

Several common ingredients in oxidation tints have proven to cause safety concerns of a variety of levels.

Recorcinol, napthas, and cocamidopropylamine are all credited with causing skin irritations. Acrylamide is toxic through skin absorption.

Morpholine can be irritating to the eyes, skin, and mucous membranes. It causes sloughing of the skin and has been associated with kidney and liver damage. Concentrated solutions of ammonium carbonate also can be irritating to the skin while ingestion causes nausea and vomiting. Intramuscular injection can be lethal. Propylene glycol is responsible for many allergic reactions and is being somewhat replaced by the safer glycols such as butylene and polyethylene glycol.

The use of 1,3-benzene in hair coloring is controversial as it is highly flammable and poisonous when ingested. It is irritating to the mucous membranes and harmful amounts may be absorbed through the skin. It can cause sensitivity to the light, which leads to rash and swelling and is believed to cause bone marrow poisoning, aplastic anemia, and leukemia. Benzene has been cited as a public health threat by several consumer safety groups and industrial regulatory agencies. In response to a petition filed by the Consumer Health Research Group, an organization affiliated with consumer advocate Ralph Nader, the Consumer Product Safety Commission voted unanimously in February of 1987 to ban the use of benzene in the manufacture of many household products. Safety standards have been set for cosmetic workers handling benzene, but it is still used in many beauty products.

Paratoluenediamine is capable of causing contact dermatitis, liver damage, and respiratory irritations. The risks involved in low level exposure are also being explored as paratoluenediamine has been discovered in the drinking water of many cities.

Paraphenylenediamine has been proven to cause skin rashes, eczema, gastritis, bronchial asthma, and on occasion, death. It can react with azo dyes and produce photosensitivity. In 1979, the National Cancer Institute reported that ingestion of some permanent hair dyes by laboratory rats led to cancer. The Food and Drug Administration announced that it could not ban the suspected hair dyes because they were exempted from such action by the 1938 Food, Drug, and Cosmetic Act. After public outcry, most manufacturers voluntarily removed 4-methoxy-m-phenylenediamine, one of the six dyes believed to cause cancer in animals. Other dyes found to penetrate human and animal skin that are associated with high risk are:

- *4-chloro-m-phenylenediamine*
- *2,4-toluenediamine*
- *2-nitro-p-phenylenediamine*
- *4-amino-2-nitrophenol*
- *2,4-diaminoanisole*

Hair coloring studies by the Chemical Workers Union and the Occupational Safety and Health Administration indicate that cosmetologists have relatively more cancers of their breasts, respiratory and digestive systems, and genital organs. One study at a major hospital shows more toxemia during pregnancy, miscarriages, premature deliveries, and smaller babies among hairdressers. A study by New York University researchers, published in the February 1987 issue of the *Journal of the National Cancer Institute,* suggests that women who have used hair dyes for more than ten years face an increased risk of developing breast cancer.

The United States, as well as many other countries, has laws requiring patch tests before using and regulations specifying the maximum concentration allowed in a formula. In the United Kingdom the Pharmacy and Poisons Act (1933) and the Poisons Rules of 1970 stipulate that all hair dyes containing phenylenediamines or tolylenediamines, or other alkylated benzene diamines or other salts must be packaged with the following warning label: "Caution. This preparation may cause serious inflammation on the skin in certain persons and should be used only in accordance with expert advice."

On April 6, 1978, the Food and Drug Administration ordered manufacturers to label permanent hair dyes with the following: "Warning. Contains an ingredient that can penetrate your skin and has been determined to cause cancer in laboratory animals." The industry successfully fought this ruling and the FDA still does not ban any ingredients in hair dyes. Even if the dye is known to cause adverse reactions under conditions of use, the product may not be considered adulterated. The FDA cannot forbid its sale and use if the label bears the following statement: "Caution. This product contains ingredients which may cause skin irritation on certain individuals, and a preliminary test according to the accompanying directions should first be made. This product must not be used for dyeing the eyelashes or eyebrows; to do so may cause blindness."

Only if the label of a color does not bear the caution statement and patch test directions may it be subjected to regulatory action if it is determined to be harmful under customary conditions of use.

Conflicting evidence and opinions have been the basis for the lack of restriction on dye ingredients. Dr. E. Cuyler Hammond, of the American Cancer Society, conducted a thirteen year test of 5,000 hairdressers and a matched group of non-hairdressers. In his study no difference was found in the two groups. Due to the still inconclusive evidence, the American Medical Association has simply offered a warning that the product be used with caution.

Even though all precautions should be observed, it is worth noting that recent technology has lately provided the industry with hair dyes having a fairly low incidence of allergic reaction. Manufacturers estimate that approximately one case of allergy occurs per 1 million units of dye applied. Improvements continue to be forthcoming with the increased purity of ingredients, improvements in the formation of products, and in the removal from the shaft of all product residue through efficient shampooing

SAFETY PRECAUTIONS FOR USE OF OXIDATION TINTS

1. Follow the Federal Food and Drug Administration guidelines for giving and interpreting a predisposition test before color application.
2. Use clean applicators, as residue from prior chemicals can adversely affect tint.
3. Do not irritate the scalp by brushing, brisk shampooing, or blow drying before application.
4. Follow all manufacturer's recommended directions.
5. Analyze hair and scalp before color application.
6. Give complete client consultation.
7. Suggest conditioning treatments if necessary.
8. Do not tint over metallic or compound dyes.
9. Perform a test strand before application to entire head.

10. Keep complete and accurate records of all chemical formulas and procedures.
11. Apply color immediately after mixing.
12. Mix in nonmetallic mixing receptacles.
13. Use a mild shampoo and cool water for product removal.
14. Protect client's clothing.
15. Do not allow product to come in contact with client's eyes.
16. Do not overlap during a retouch application.
17. Wash hands before and after each client and observe all sanitation regulations.
18. Wear gloves to protect your hands from stains, chemical burns, and the possibility of allergy and absorption through the skin.
19. Do not save left over product. It can swell, causing the top to explode off the applicator bottle or product to run over the side of the bowl.
20. Never use tint on the eyelashes or eyebrows. **To do so may cause blindness.**

COLOR SELECTION

Color selection in oxidation tints is never an absolute, as color results are affected by the condition, texture, and porosity of the hair as well as by prior chemical services and the room temperature. However, the following guidelines will lead the way to the selection of formulas appropriate for performing a test strand.

Tinting Darker

Tinting darker is the addition of artificial pigment to natural pigment. The artificial pigment causes the hair to absorb more light and reflect less, thus creating a color that the eye perceives as darker. The fact that "color on color creates a darker color" often leads to hues that are darker than pictured on the color chart. Generally it is advisable to select a shade that is a ½ level lighter than the desired final results.

If the hair is porous the color will process quicker and darker than intended by the manufacturer and create a darker color than on nonporous hair. If the hair is slightly porous, select a color that is 1 level lighter than desired in the finished results. If the hair is very porous, select a color that is 1 to 2 levels lighter than desired in the finished results.

Use the Chromatic Circle to adjust hue and saturation.

Tinting Lighter

Use the following formula for color selection when lightening:

FORMULATION STEP	EXAMPLE
1. Identify the desired level.	5
2. Identify the natural level.	−3
3. Subtract the natural level from the desired level.	2
4. Add the level difference to the desired level.	+5
5. The total is the level of color needed.	7

Any total that is over 10 indicates that either a higher level of H_2O_2 or prelightening is necessary to achieve the desired level. Lifting more than two levels causes warm off-tones that will need to be neutralized with the tone selection of the hue. Use the Chromatic Circle as a reference.

THE SOAP CAP

A soap cap is the addition of equal amounts of shampoo to tint solution to create a milder formula. This technique is used in several different hair coloring procedures.

The most common use of a soap cap is to refresh color on the ends of the hair during a tint retouch service. However, it is an optional procedure. Whether or not the hair requires a soap cap is determined by the colorist during the client consultation.

All oxidation tints fade in between monthly retouch services due to alkaline shampoos, exposure to the elements, other chemical services, and various styling tools and techniques. When the hair fades or goes off-tone enough that there is an obvious difference between the fresh color and the old, a soap cap is recommended to blend the color from scalp to ends.

However, if the color hue, level, and saturation have not changed since the last color service, no soap cap is necessary and may even be harmful. Depositing artificial color molecules on top of artificial color molecules creates a *darker color*. Therefore, if the soap cap is done unnecessarily, the ends of the hair will turn darker and darker with each subsequent retouch service.

If a lightening product is soap capped through the ends excessively the color can become over-lightened. In this case the ends of the hair strands will begin to absorb the color too quickly and process off-tone.

Unnecessary soap caps will also increase the porosity of the hair and lead to excessive damage to the hair strands. The formulation of a soap cap creates a solution that is milder than the mixture applied at the scalp, but it is still quite strong and alkaline in reaction.

A soap cap is created after the processing time on the scalp is complete. At this time the colorist adds equal amounts of shampoo to the leftover tint and stirs it thoroughly. The mixture is applied quickly and worked gently through the ends of the hair. If the hair is strong and in good condition, a tint comb is used to ensure complete blending of the color. If the hair is very weak or fragile, the product is not combed through the hair because the tension on hair in a weakened alkaline state could cause loss of strength, elasticity, or even breakage. Bleach is never soap capped or combed through the ends on a retouch service because it creates an extremely soft condition during the processing stage. A chemical haircut would almost certainly result from combing bleach through the hair.

The timing of a soap cap is generally very short in comparison with the timing of the undiluted product at the scalp. The hair receiving the soap cap has received prior coloring treatments; therefore, the color processes very quickly. Approximately 10 minutes or less is the average time a soap cap is allowed to remain on the ends.

Occasionally a soap cap is used between tint retouches to freshen the color. However, this is done only for emergency reasons. Two serious problems can result from soap capping between tint retouches. The first is that the hair becomes more porous from the application of this alkaline solution. The second problem occurs if the virgin hair has grown out enough to be noticeable at the scalp. This resistant hair will not process to the same color as the previously tinted ends. This can result in the need for corrective coloring, which is time consuming and costly for the client.

A soap cap is also used in conjunction with a tint back to natural service if the tint does not exactly match the natural color. A quick soap cap will break the line of demarcation when the colorist determines that it is necessary.

LEVEL 1—BLACK OXIDATION TINT COMPARISON

EXPERIMENT INSTRUCTION SHEET

Objectives

To observe and document the results of application of the same black oxidation tint on four different levels of natural hair color. To gain experience mixing oxidation tints.

Hair Swatches Needed

4 virgin hair swatches of the following color levels:

- Level 2—Dark brown
- Level 4—Light brown
- Level 6—Dark blonde
- Level 8—Light blonde

Labeling Hair Swatches

Label each swatch as to the level of its natural color.

Materials Needed

- Level 1—Black tint
- 20 volume hydrogen peroxide
- Nonmetallic mixing receptacle

Product Formulation

1. Place 1 teaspoon of black tint in a nonmetallic mixing receptacle.
2. Mix in the appropriate amount of 20 volume hydrogen peroxide.

Procedure

1. Apply the black tint mixture to all swatches.
2. Processs at room temperature for 40 minutes.
3. Rinse, shampoo, dry.
4. Mount swatches on the *Experiment Results Sheet on page R-53.*
5. Answer *Review Questions on page R-55.*

LEVEL 3—MEDIUM BROWN OXIDATION TINT COMPARISON

EXPERIMENT INSTRUCTION SHEET

Objectives

To observe and document the results of application of the same brown oxidation tint on four different levels of natural hair color. To gain experience mixing oxidation tints.

Hair Swatches Needed

4 virgin hair swatches of the following color levels:

- Level 2—Dark brown
- Level 4—Light brown
- Level 6—Dark blonde
- Level 8—Light blonde

Labeling Hair Swatches

Label each swatch as to the level of its natural color.

Materials Needed

- Level 3—Medium brown tint
- 20 volume hydrogen peroxide
- Nonmetallic mixing receptacle

Product Formulation

1. Place 1 teaspoon of brown tint in a nonmetallic mixing receptacle.
2. Mix in the appropriate amount of 20 volume hydrogen peroxide.

Procedure

1. Apply the brown tint mixture to all swatches.
2. Processs at room temperature for 40 minutes.
3. Rinse, shampoo, dry.
4. Mount swatches on the *Experiment Results Sheet on page R-57.*
5. Answer *Review Questions on page R-59.*

LEVEL 7—MEDIUM BLONDE OXIDATION TINT COMPARISON

EXPERIMENT INSTRUCTION SHEET

Objectives

To observe and document the results of application of the same blonde oxidation tint on four different levels of natural hair color. To gain experience mixing oxidation tints.

Hair Swatches Needed

4 virgin hair swatches of the following color levels:

- Level 2—Dark brown
- Level 4—Light brown
- Level 6—Dark blonde
- Level 8—Light blonde

Labeling Hair Swatches

Label each swatch as to the level of its natural color.

Materials Needed

- Level 7—Medium blonde tint
- 20 volume hydrogen peroxide
- Nonmetallic mixing receptacle

Product Formulation

1. Place 1 teaspoon of blonde tint in a nonmetallic mixing receptacle.
2. Mix in the appropriate amount of 20 volume hydrogen peroxide.

Procedure

1. Apply the blonde tint mixture to all swatches.
2. Process at room temperature for 40 minutes.
3. Rinse, shampoo, dry.
4. Mount swatches on the *Experiment Results Sheet on page R-61.*
5. Answer *Review Questions on page R-63.*

LEVEL 10—LIGHTEST BLONDE TINTS

EXPERIMENT INSTRUCTION SHEET

Objectives

To observe and document the level of lift when using the lightest blonde tints on four different levels of natural hair color. To gain experience mixing oxidation tints.

Hair Swatches Needed

4 virgin hair swatches of the following color levels:

- Level 2—Dark brown
- Level 4—Light brown
- Level 6—Dark blonde
- Level 8—Light blonde

Labeling Hair Swatches

Label each swatch as to the level of its natural color.

Materials Needed

- Level 10—Lightest blonde
- 20 volume hydrogen peroxide
- Nonmetallic mixing receptacle

Product Formulation

1. Place 1 teaspoon of blonde tint in a nonmetallic mixing receptacle.
2. Mix in the appropriate amount of 20 volume hydrogen peroxide.

Procedure

1. Apply the lightest blonde tint mixture to all swatches.
2. Processs at room temperature for 40 minutes.
3. Rinse, shampoo, dry.
4. Mount swatches on the *Experiment Results Sheet on page R-65.*
5. Answer *Review Questions on page R-67*

5

Hydrogen Peroxide

Hydrogen peroxide was discovered in 1818 by a Frenchman named Louis Thenard. In addition to its role in hair coloring, the versatile hydrogen peroxide has many other important uses, depending upon its strength. Solutions of 90 percent or greater concentrations were used after World War II to provide oxygen to burn the fuel in submarine engines. A solution of 30 percent is used to bleach ivory, wool, cotton, silk, straw, and feathers. A 3 percent solution serves as a disinfectant and a mouth wash. A variety of strengths are sometimes found on the ingredients list of permanent wave neutralizers. Hydrogen peroxide is also used seasonally in Bournemouth and Poole, England and all year round in Texas, U.S.A. to combat the odors in sewers.

CHEMICAL COMPOSITION OF HYDROGEN PEROXIDE

Pure hydrogen peroxide is a colorless liquid with unpredictable and explosive properties that make it dangerous to work with. The chemical formula for this compound is H_2O_2. This means that hydrogen peroxide is made up of two atoms of oxygen for each two atoms of hydrogen.

When hydrogen and oxygen combine spontaneously they form water (H_2O), which is a stable compound, unlikely to change its form. However, hydrogen peroxide, as a manmade rather than a natural compound, is unstable due to the forced addition of oxygen. An uncapped bottle allows the extra, unstable oxygen atom to escape, thus turning the hydrogen peroxide (H_2O_2) back into water (H_2O).

Contrary to popular belief, when the top is removed from the bottle and a "pop" is heard, the product is getting weaker rather than maintaining its strength. The "pop" is the oxygen gas being set free prematurely.

Occasionally, a bottle of peroxide will bulge, particularly at the bottom so that the bottle cannot set flat. This indicates that the oxygen atoms are escaping from the hydrogen peroxide and building up pressure within the container. A bottle distorted in this way must be opened with caution because the liquid may shoot out as the oxygen atoms make a violent escape.

In its pure form, hydrogen peroxide has a pH of approximately 7.0. Diluted with water and other additives as produced for use by hair colorists, it falls within the "mild" acidic pH range of 3.5 to 4.0.

Most hydrogen peroxide solutions are packaged in opaque bottles because light causes them to break down rapidly. Heat has the same effect. Therefore, the manufacturers recommend storage in a dark, cool area. If stored safely, a stabilized, uncontaminated bottle, either partially or completely full, is expected to retain its quality for up to three years.

ACTION OF HYDROGEN PEROXIDE

Hydrogen peroxide serves as the oxidizing agent most commonly used in cosmetology. An oxidizer is defined as a substance that causes oxygen to combine with another substance, such as melanin. After oxygen and melanin have combined, the peroxide solution begins to diffuse (break apart and spread out) the melanin within the hair shaft. This diffused or shattered pigment is characteristic of hair that has a light appearance to the eye. This diffused melanin is now called oxymelanin.

This degree of lightening is relatively mild and causes little damage to the hair shaft. If pale, delicate shades are desired, this degree of lightening is not sufficient and the hair must be further lightened.

The oxymelanin molecule is difficult to oxidize further. The molecule must be totally diffused to achieve a lighter shade. This requires that the treatment be left on for a longer period of time, or a stronger formula used such as a peroxide solution containing sodium persulfate, potassium persulfate, urea peroxide, and/or ammonia.

TYPES OF HYDROGEN PEROXIDE

Hydrogen peroxide is distributed by manufacturers under a variety of names: *developer, oxidizer, generator,* and *catalyst* just to name a few. (Some manufacturers also use the word "catalyst" to mean *protinator.*) However, regardless of which name is used, only three basic classifications of hydrogen peroxide exist: *dry, cream,* and *liquid.*

Dry Hydrogen Peroxide

Dry hydrogen peroxide is generally available in tablet form for use with oxidation tints. The tablet is dissolved in liquid hydrogen peroxide to boost its volume and then mixed with the color. The availability of liquid peroxides in a variety of volumes has made this product somewhat obsolete.

Cream Hydrogen Peroxide

Cream peroxides contain several additives such as thickeners, drabbers, conditioners (lanolin type), urea, and an acid for stabilization. Cream peroxide tends to create a thick, creamy formula that is easy to control and, therefore, is often called the "stay put" peroxide. This extra control helps to prevent dripping during the use of the brush and bowl method of application. This thicker formula is also advantageous when used in foil-wrap weaving, hair painting, or frosting because the bleach is less likely to "bleed" onto places where it is not wanted. The creamy formula also tends to stay moist on the hair longer than liquid peroxide.

However, cream peroxide cannot be used with every oxidation product. Because of the additives and its extra thickness, cream peroxide is not compatible in all bleaching and tinting formulas. Also, the additive of cream peroxide often creates a solution that is not strong enough to offer complete coverage when coloring gray hair. Always check the manufacturer's directions before mixing to determine if this peroxide with all its additives is the one recommended for use with that particular product.

Chemical Composition of Cream Hydrogen Peroxide

Acetic acid is commonly used in cream peroxides as a pH adjuster. This clear, colorless liquid is also used in hand lotions, permanent dyes, and as a solvent for gums and resins. Acetic acid occurs naturally in a variety of citrus and non-citrus fruits, cheese, coffee, and skimmed milk. Vinegar is about 4-6 percent acetic acid.

Phosphoric acid is another of the acids used as a pH adjuster. It doubles as an anti-oxidant and is popular in cream peroxides because it mixes easily with both the water and alcohol, which are also regularly found on the ingredients list.

Ceteth-2, technically known as polyethylene (2) cetyl ether, is a compound of the derivatives of a variety of alcohols. It is mixed with a gas that works as a fungicide and a wetting agent that allows the product to spread more thoroughly on the hair shaft.

Nonoxynol, or *polyoxyethylene nonyl phenyl ether*, as it is chemically known, is added to cream peroxides as a nonionic surface-acting surfactant. The nonionic qualities of this chemical help to prevent freezing and shrinking of the product. Surface-active surfactant means that this ingredient, like ceteth-2, is a wetting agent that allows the peroxide to spread out and penetrate easier.

Oleamide (oleamide DEA, oleylamide, or oleic acid) is an oil obtained from animal and vegetable fats. It helps to prevent excessive drying of the hair and gives the product a slightly thicker consistency. Oleamide is also used in permanent wave solution, cold cream, nail polish, shampoo, liquid makeup, and lipstick.

Cetyl alcohol is an emollient that, if the concentration is strong enough, can leave a smooth, slick coating on the hair that improves its appearance and manageability after the hair color service is complete. It is widely used in cosmetics such as lipstick, mascara, cream rouge and hair products such as straightener, lacquer, hairdressing, and shampoo. It is occasionally added to the ingredient list of laxatives. Cetyl alcohol is made from a wax that is derived from the head tissues of the sperm whale.

Stearyl alcohol, prepared from sperm whale oil, is also a common ingredient in cream peroxides as well as in cosmetics, hair rinses, shampoos and depilatories.

Glycerine is a by-product of the manufacturing process of soap. It absorbs moisture from the air and helps to keep the product from drying out even if the user forgets to put the lid back on the container. Glycerine also helps cream peroxide spread better. It is used as a humectant in food, skin freshener, mouthwashes, facial products, and toothpastes.

Sodium stannate is a white or colorless inorganic salt. It serves as a humectant in hair dyes and cream peroxides and is similar in action to glycerine.

Acetanilid or *acetanilide*, made from aniline and acetic acid, is used for its ability to give an opaque mat finish. It was first used as a coal tar analgesic and anti-fever agent. However, it is not widely used today because related products with less toxicity now are available.

Pentasodium pentetate, sodium tripolyphosphate (STPP), pentapotassium triphosphate, pentasodium triphosphate, or pentasodium diethylenetriaminepentaacetate, is an inorganic salt that works as a dispersing agent, emulsifier, and a preservative to prevent both physical and chemical changes that would affect the color, texture, and appearance of the oxidation dyes. It is also used in cleansing creams and cosmetic lotions.

Tetrasodium pyrophosphate (TSPP) works as an emulsifier so that the cream peroxide does not separate and need to be shaken before addition to the dye.

Oxyquinoline sulfate is added to cream peroxide for its ability to prevent fungus growth and act as a preservative. It is a white crystal or powder that does not dissolve easily in water unless alcohol, acetone, or benzene is also present.

Liquid Hydrogen Peroxide

Clear liquid peroxide does not contain any additives other than a stabilizing acid. Acids stabilize peroxide through the ability to form hydrogen ions when dissolved in water. A variety of acids are available for use as acid adjusters or pH balancers.

Citric acid (vitamin C) is widely used in hydrogen peroxide as well as many other cosmetics to lower alkalinity. This is the same vitamin that is a well-known nutrient supplement.

Phosphate is an acid adjuster that has the advantage of also working as an anti-oxidant. Phosphate is a salt derived from phosphoric acid, which is made from phosphate rock. It can be used as an emulsifier, texturizer, and a sequestrant in both cosmetics and foods.

Liquid peroxide is convenient because it can be used in *almost* every bleach and tint formula on the market today. Another plus is that the formula for liquid peroxide is basically the same from one manufacturer to another rather than varied as with the cream peroxide. This offers the colorist consistency of coloring results regardless of the brand of hydrogen peroxide used. The lack of additives in liquid hydrogen peroxide creates a color formula that generally covers gray effectively.

The minuses to be considered in choosing liquid peroxide over cream are that the bleaches and dyes tend to dry out faster, and the conditioning agents are not present. However, one peroxide is not superior to the other. They are just different. It is the responsibility of the colorist to read the manufacturer's recommended directions and select the "best" product for the job.

Strengths of Hydrogen Peroxide

Both the cream and liquid forms of hydrogen peroxide are available in a variety of strengths. Scientists identify the different strengths by percentages such as 3 percent and 6 percent. Cosmetologists identify the various strengths by volume because it is the "freeing" of a certain volume of gases that creates the desired chemical reaction in hair coloring. Note the comparison of the two methods of identifying the strengths of hydrogen peroxide:

Percentage of H_2O_2 in water—	1.5%	3%	6%	9%	15%	30%
Volume of oxygen to be set free—	5	10	20	30	50	100

With the following formulas, the colorist can calculate either the percentage or volume of any strength of hydrogen peroxide. To calculate the percentage of peroxide if the volume is known, compute: Volume × .3 = % of the H_2O_2. To calculate the volume if the percentage is known, compute: 10 × % divided by 3 = volume. (Do not change the % to a decimal.)

As the volumes of oxygen gas in any strength of hydrogen peroxide are set free, it reverts to water. This is considered an advantage because no dangerous residue is formed and left behind to damage the hair.

SAFETY

The majority of the additives in hydrogen peroxide are considered nontoxic and nonharmful in the strengths used. For example, in a concentrated form acetic acid is highly corrosive and capable of causing lung damage. However, less than 5 percent solutions are considered safe and can only cause a mild irritation on the skin.

Oleamide possesses low oral toxicity and can be mildly irritating to the skin. Glycerine, in strong solutions, can be irritating to mucous membranes, but as used by the cosmetic industry it is considered nontoxic, nonirritating, and nonallergenic.

Acetanilid is no longer extensively used in the formulation of hydrogen peroxides because it can cause eczema when applied to the skin. In tests where rats were fed doses of 3500 milligrams per kilogram of body weight, tumors were caused.

STPP in concentrated solutions is only moderately irritating to the skin, but ingestion causes violent vomiting. Therefore, it is advisable to keep this solution out of the hands of children.

Twenty volume or 6 percent hydrogen peroxide is the strength recommended by manufacturers for use with most bleaches and oxidation tints. While the vapor from the use of stronger levels of hydrogen peroxide is harmless, if not handled properly, the more concentrated solutions can cause skin irritation, chemical burns, and hair damage. It is especially risky to mix the higher levels of hydrogen peroxide with bleach formulated for use with 20 volume because the ingredients in the product itself, such as boosters, activators, or protinators, also work to increase the strength of the formula. However, a volume lower than 20 will not release enough oxygen to lighten the hair properly.

Volumes as great as 130 percent are packaged for purchase and use by the cosmetologist. This strength creates a highly volatile and potentially dangerous material if not used with care. While any hydrogen peroxide of strength of 20 or higher volume can cause chemical burns, the possibility and severity increase in proportion to the strength of the peroxide. Twenty volume generally does no noticeable damage if it is rinsed off the skin quickly. At the other end of the spectrum, 130 volume becomes caustic immediately upon contact with skin and mucous membranes.

Contamination

The slightest amount of impurity in a developer may cause tint or lightener to froth. This frothing can cause uneven application and color results. Contaminated 20 volume hydrogen peroxide will also fail to lighten the hair properly. Once hydrogen peroxide is poured from its original container, it should not be returned to that or another stock bottle. Contact with dust in the air or any organic material will contaminate the hydrogen peroxide and cause it to break down rapidly. Inconsistent and unpredictable color results from this weakening of the working power of the product.

Contact with metals or metallic salts has the opposite, yet also adverse, reaction on hydrogen peroxide. Contact with any metal should be avoided whether from metallic hair coloring products, a metal clip, or mixing bowl. Metal speeds up the release of the oxygen molecules and can cause hydrogen peroxide to oxidize the product before it can penetrate the cuticle and cortical layers to reach the melanin.

Use of Gloves

While hydrogen peroxide itself generally has no incidence of allergic reaction, nor does it stain the skin, it does have the ability to destroy protein and cause itching, burning, and damage to living tissues. Therefore, the use of gloves is recommended. If hydrogen peroxide accidentally gets inside a glove, do not allow it to remain in between the glove and the skin. Body heat increases the action of the hydrogen peroxide and the degree of chemical burn to the skin.

HYDROMETER

The hydrometer is used to measure the volume of liquid hydrogen peroxide. The hydrometer measures the volumes of liquid peroxide by identifying the "specific gravity" of the solution. Specific gravity tells how the density of any substance compares to the density of water. In other words it compares the weight of the liquid hydrogen peroxide to the weight of water.

The hydrometer does not measure the volume of cream peroxide because a great number of its additives are denser than water. Creams can be measured for their specific gravity, or how much denser than water they are, but this does not indicate the volumes as it does in liquid peroxide.

The colorist can use the hydrometer in several ways. First, it can be used to simply check the volume of a packaged liquid peroxide to affirm its strength. Occasionally a cap is left off or a product gets pushed to the back of a shelf, and it is best not to "assume" it is still potent.

Secondly, the hydrometer can be a money saving device. It is more economical to purchase the higher volume and dilute it in the salon than to buy an equivalent of prepackaged lower volumes.

Thirdly, the versatility and availability of all volumes of peroxide can stimulate creativity and provide the resources necessary to solve many hair coloring problems.

The hydrometer is used outside of the beauty industry in hospitals to test sediment in urine, in fish aquariums to measure the amount of salt, and in ceramic and porcelain manufacture to test product thickness.

The hydrometer looks much like a thermometer and must be handled in much the same way. It is quite delicate. It must be handled and stored carefully to prevent breakage.

HOW TO MEASURE AND ADJUST VOLUMES OF HYDROGEN PEROXIDE

Materials Needed

- Distilled water
- Nonmetallic stir stick
- Hydrometer

- Paper towels
- Gloves
- 130 volume liquid hydrogen peroxide
- Beaker
- Empty nonmetallic container
- Marking pen
- Protective apron

Table Set-Up

1. Work near running water in case any chemicals come in contact with skin.
2. Cover work area with paper towels.
3. All containers should be distinctly marked with the label facing the operator.
4. Operator's hands, beaker, hydrometer, and container for newly mixed peroxide must be thoroughly washed and dried to avoid contamination of products.
5. Place the beaker on top of the paper towels to prevent spillage from running down counter.

Procedure Measuring Existing Volumes

1. Pour H_2O_2 into beaker.
2. Slip hydrometer gently into beaker. Do not let go until you feel it begin to float. If it hits the bottom of the beaker, either or both may break.
3. When the floating hydrometer stops bobbing, read volumes on the hydrometer at the waterline.

Adjusting Volumes

1. To reduce volumes, add distilled water, stir, and read the hydrometer at the waterline.
2. To increase volumes, add hydrogen peroxide of a greater volume than that being created, stir, and read the hydrometer at the waterline.

Storage

1. Remove hydrometer, rinse, dry, and store safely.
2. Pour newly mixed hydrogen peroxide from beaker into clean container.
3. Cap tightly.
4. Rinse outside of bottle and dry.
5. Mark contents of new bottle with volumes and date.
6. Store in a cool, dark, low shelf.

Storage and Safety Rules

1. Store in a cool, dark cabinet. A low cabinet is safer than a high one to prevent spillage on colorist.
2. Point the lid away when opening.
3. Immediately flood the skin or eyes with water upon contact. Chemical burns or blindness may result.

4. Thoroughly clean area after use. Hydrogen peroxide looks like water.
5. When using over 20 volume peroxide, rinse off outside of bottle to prevent contact burns.
6. Never use more than 10 volume or 3 percent hydrogen peroxide on the skin.
7. Wear rubber gloves.
8. Touching the mouth of the container will contaminate the entire bottle.
9. Do not pour leftover hydrogen peroxide back into original or any other storage container. It will be contaminated by contact with dirt, dust, residue of prior chemicals, metals, and organic materials.
10. Do not replace the original lid with a cork. Cork is an organic substance that will cause the peroxide to lose its strength.
11. Dilute hydrogen peroxide with distilled, purified, or de-ionized water.
12. Drying 130 volume peroxide on clothing or other combustible materials may cause a fire.
13. In case of fire, use water.
14. Allow no smoking or use of any open fire or spark near hydrogen peroxide, especially the higher volumes.

USES OF HIGH AND LOW VOLUME HYDROGEN PEROXIDE

The higher the volume of hydrogen peroxide, the more diffusion of melanin. Technology has shown how high volumes of peroxide can be utilized to achieve stages of lightening that previously could only be achieved with bleach.

The lower the volume of hydrogen peroxide, the less diffusion of melanin within the hair shaft. This means that it is now possible to deposit artificial pigment into the cortex with limited diffusion of natural color while causing limited damage and change to the structure of the hair.

The unnecessary diffusion of melanin and its change into oxymelanin is responsible for the unwanted brassy tones that appear as dark tint begins to fade. The use of low volume hydrogen peroxide avoids this problem.

Use of low volume hydrogen peroxide is suggested any time it is desirable to gently deposit color without lift. The fact that low volume peroxide does less damage to the hair shaft is also valuable when toning highly bleached hair that needs no further diffusion of color.

**LEVEL 10 — BLONDE TINT
FORMULATED WITH HIGH AND LOW VOLUME H$_2$O$_2$**

EXPERIMENT INSTRUCTION SHEET

Objectives

To observe and document the color results when using different volumes of hydrogen peroxide in standard tint formulas. To gain experience mixing and formulating with 10, 20, 30, and 40 volumes of hydrogen peroxide.

Hair Swatches Needed

4 virgin hair swatches of either of the following color levels:

- Level 7—medium blonde
- Level 8—light blonde

Labeling Hair Swatches

Label swatches as follows:

- 10 volume
- 20 volume
- 30 volume
- 40 volume

Materials Needed

- Level 10—Lightest blonde permanent tint
- Hydrogen peroxide—10, 20, 30, and 40 volumes
- Nonmetallic mixing receptacles

Formulation

1. *Swatch #1*—Mix 1 teaspoon of tint with the appropriate amount of 10 volume hydrogen peroxide in nonmetallic mixing receptacle.
2. *Swatch #2*—Mix 1 teaspoon of tint with the appropriate amount of 20 volume hydrogen peroxide in nonmetallic mixing receptacle.
3. *Swatch #3*—Mix 1 teaspoon of tint with the appropriate amount of 30 volume hydrogen peroxide in nonmetallic mixing receptacle.
4. *Swatch #4*—Mix 1 teaspoon of tint with the appropriate amount of 40 volume hydrogen peroxide in nonmetallic mixing receptacle.

Procedure

1. Apply each formulation to the appropriately marked swatch.
2. Process at room temperature for 40 minutes.
3. Rinse with cool water, shampoo, and dry.
4. Mount swatches on the *Experiment Results Sheet on page R-69.*
5. Answer *Review Questions on page R-71.*

**LEVEL 5 — AUBURN TINT
FORMULATED WITH HIGH AND LOW VOLUME H$_2$O$_2$**

EXPERIMENT INSTRUCTION SHEET

Objectives

To observe and document the color results when using different volumes of hydrogen peroxide in standard tint formulas. To gain experience mixing and formulating with 10, 20, 30, and 40 volumes of hydrogen peroxide.

Hair Swatches Needed

4 virgin hair swatches of either of the following color levels:

- Level 5—Lightest brown
- Level 6—Dark blonde

Labeling Hair Swatches

Label swatches as follows:

- 10 volume
- 20 volume
- 30 volume
- 40 volume

Materials Needed

- Level 5—Auburn permanent tint
- Hydrogen peroxide—10, 20, 30, and 40 volumes
- Nonmetallic mixing receptacles

Formulation

1. *Swatch #1*—Mix 1 teaspoon of tint with the appropriate amount of 10 volume hydrogen peroxide in nonmetallic mixing receptacle.
2. *Swatch #2*—Mix 1 teaspoon of tint with the appropriate amount of 20 volume hydrogen peroxide in nonmetallic mixing receptacle.
3. *Swatch #3*—Mix 1 teaspoon of tint with the appropriate amount of 30 volume hydrogen peroxide in nonmetallic mixing receptacle.
4. *Swatch #4*—Mix 1 teaspoon of tint with the appropriate amount of 40 volume hydrogen peroxide in nonmetallic mixing receptacle.

Procedure

1. Apply each formulation to the appropriately marked swatch.
2. Process at room temperature for 40 minutes.
3. Rinse with cool water, shampoo, and dry.
4. Mount swatches on the *Experiment Results Sheet on page R-73*.
5. Answer *Review Questions on page R-75*.

LEVEL 3 — BROWN TINT
FORMULATED WITH HIGH AND LOW VOLUME H$_2$O$_2$

EXPERIMENT INSTRUCTION SHEET

Objectives

To observe and document the color results when using different volumes of hydrogen peroxide in standard tint formulas. To gain experience mixing and formulating with 10, 20, 30, and 40 volumes of hydrogen peroxide.

Hair Swatches Needed

4 virgin hair swatches of either of the following color levels:

- Level 3—Medium brown
- Level 4—Light brown

Labeling Hair Swatches

Label swatches as follows:

- 10 volume
- 20 volume
- 30 volume
- 40 volume

Materials Needed

- Level 3—Medium brown permanent tint
- Hydrogen peroxide—10, 20, 30, and 40 volumes
- Nonmetallic mixing receptacles

Formulation

1. *Swatch #1*—Mix 1 teaspoon of tint with the appropriate amount of 10 volume hydrogen peroxide in nonmetallic mixing receptacle.
2. *Swatch #2*—Mix 1 teaspoon of tint with the appropriate amount of 20 volume hydrogen peroxide in nonmetallic mixing receptacle.

3. *Swatch #3*—Mix 1 teaspoon of tint with the appropriate amount of 30 volume hydrogen peroxide in nonmetallic mixing receptacle.
4. *Swatch #4*—Mix 1 teaspoon of tint with the appropriate amount of 40 volume hydrogen peroxide in nonmetallic mixing receptacle.

Procedure

1. Apply each formulation to the appropriately marked swatch.
2. Process at room temperature for 40 minutes.
3. Rinse with cool water, shampoo, and dry.
4. Mount swatches on the *Experiment Results Sheet on page R-77.*
5. Answer *Review Questions on page R-79.*

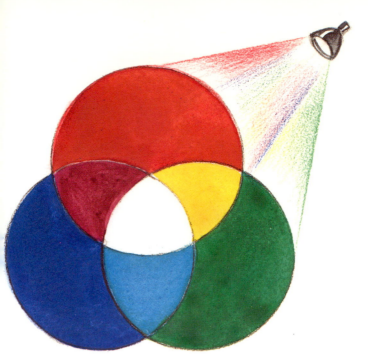

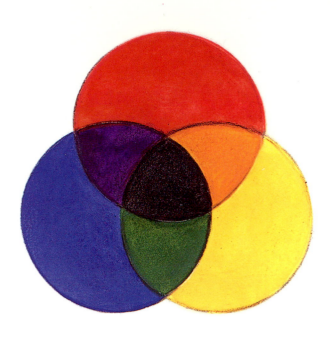

Plate 1. Additive Color Mixing. Beaming one colored light from the spectrum on top of another adds one color to the other, creating a new color.

Plate 2. Subtractive Color Mixing. The addition of more colors to a mixture subtracts the amount of white light that is reflected to the eye.

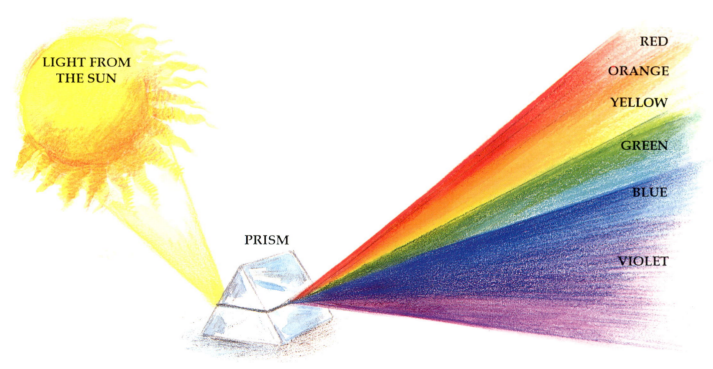

LIGHT FROM
THE SUN

PRISM

RED

ORANGE

YELLOW

GREEN

BLUE

VIOLET

Plate 3. The white light of the sun is a blending of all the colors of the spectrum. A prism separates the colors by bending them through different angles. The beam of separated colored lights, arranged in order from violet to red, is called the spectrum of the sunlight.

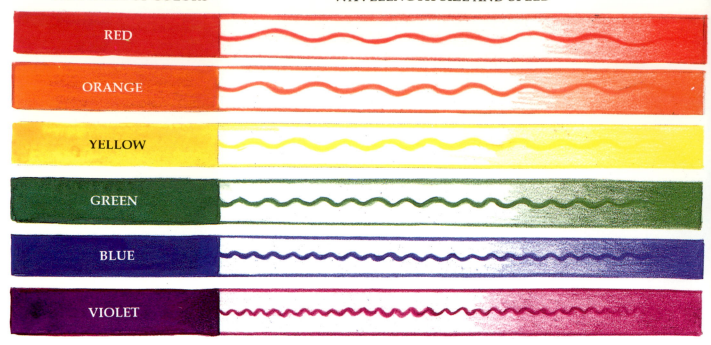

SPECTRUM OF COLORS   **WAVELENGTH SIZE AND SPEED**

RED

ORANGE

YELLOW

GREEN

BLUE

VIOLET

Plate 4. What makes the separate colored beams in the spectrum different is the fact that they differ in size and speed. Waves of red light are the longest and slowest. Waves of violet are the shortest and quickest.

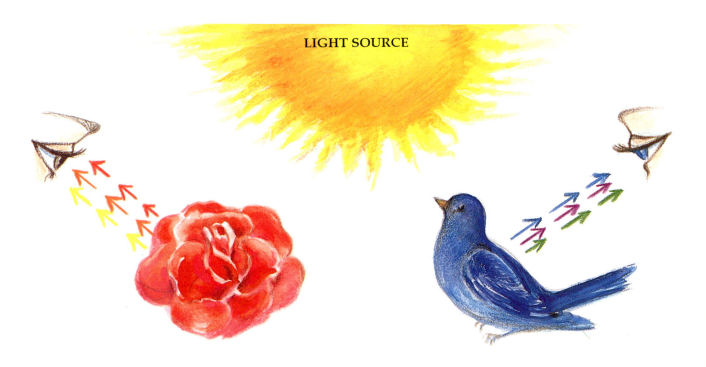

LIGHT SOURCE

Plate 5. On a surface known as red, a beam of white light strikes a red surface. The pigment molecules in the surface selectively absorb all the short wavelengths and reflect the long rays to the eyes. A blue surface absorbs long and medium waves. Short lightwaves are reflected to produce the sensation of blue.

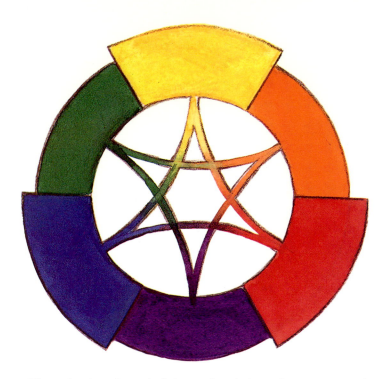

Plate 6. A color triad is made of three hues an equal distance apart on the Chromatic Circle. Connecting lines to form a triangle point out the three colors of a triad. When combined in a variety of levels and saturations, the hues in a triad generally are pleasing to the eye.

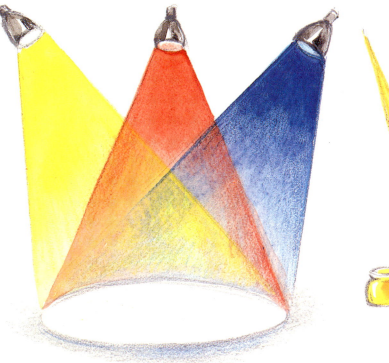

Plate 7. Additive Color Mixing. Combining light rays of all the primary colors creates white light.

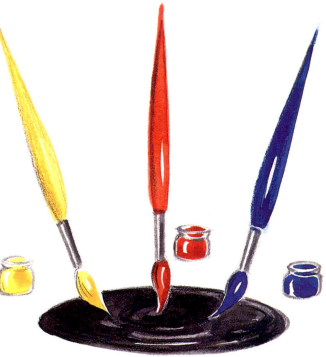

Plate 8. Subtractive Color Mixing. Combining pigments of all pure primary colors creates black.

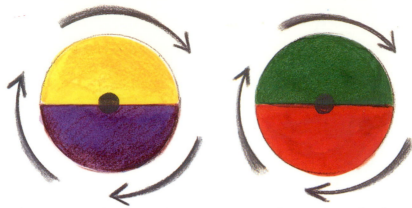

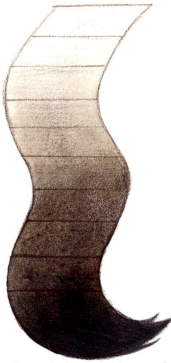

Plate 9. Complementary hues are positioned opposite each other on the Chromatic Circle. Together they contain the complete spectrum of hue. If you put complementary colors on a wheel and spin it very rapidly, the colors will "blend" to gray.

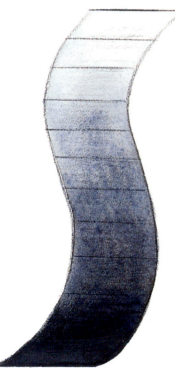

Plate 10. Neutralizing pure true colors creates the neutral shades that range from lightest gray to black.

Plate 11. Neutralizing balanced colors such as hair coloring products creates the neutral shades of beige to black.

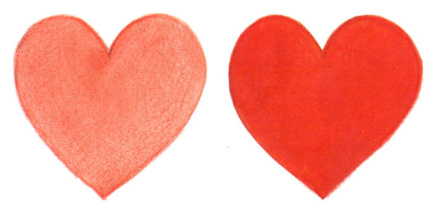

Plate 12. Red can be red, or it can be vividly red!

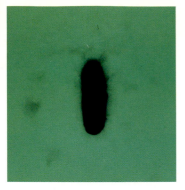

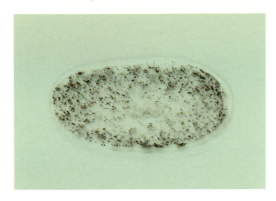

Plate 14. A cross-section of ethnic black hair showing the large amount of melanin in the cortex. *(Courtesy: Redken Laboratories, Inc.)*

Plate 13. Technology now provides microscopes that are so powerful that they can see inside a hair shaft. This picture of a single oval-shaped, blackish brown melanin molecule is the basis for all hair color. The green is a chemical used by the scientist to mount the molecule on the slide. *(Courtesy: Redken Laboratories, Inc.)*

Plate 15. Almost nonexistent melanin molecule of virgin gray hair. *(Courtesy: Redken Laboratories, Inc.)*

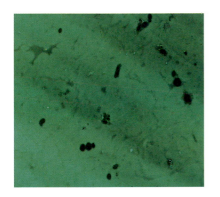

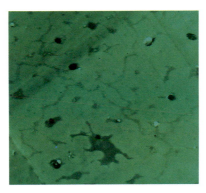

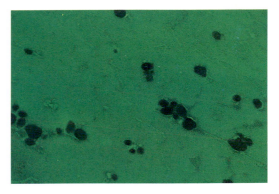

Plate 16. Virgin blonde hair contains relatively small molecular size with lesser amounts distributed throughout the length of the cortex. The empty spaces are air pockets. *(Courtesy: Redken Laboratories, Inc.).*

Plate 17. This molecular distribution of slightly larger molecules is characteristic of virgin light red hair. *(Courtesy: Redken Laboratories, Inc.)*

Plate 18. Virgin brown hair typically contains a greater number of melanin molecules of varying sizes. *(Courtesy: Redken Laboratories, Inc.)*

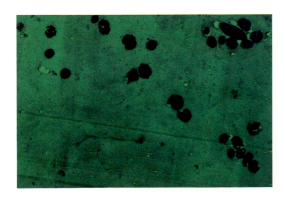

Plate 19. Virgin black hair contains the greatest number of melanin molecules. While the molecules vary in size, just as in the other colors, black hair typically has the greatest number of large molecules, causing a greater absorption of light rays. As we know from the Laws of Color, the absorption of all speeds and lengths of light rays creates a lack of reflection. We describe this phenomena of selective absorption and reflection as color. This particular arrangement of pigment we have named "black." *(Courtesy: Redken Laboratories, Inc.)*

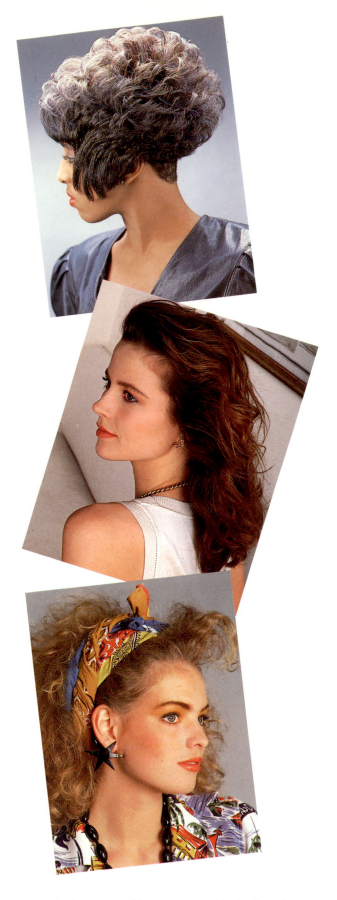

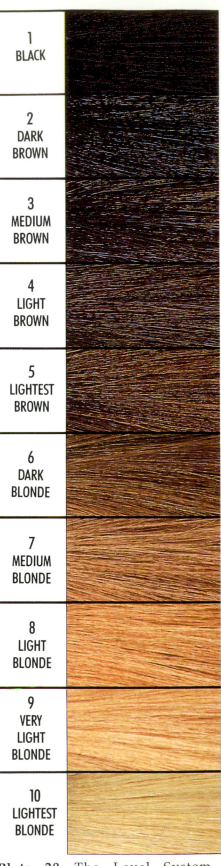

1	BLACK
2	DARK BROWN
3	MEDIUM BROWN
4	LIGHT BROWN
5	LIGHTEST BROWN
6	DARK BLONDE
7	MEDIUM BLONDE
8	LIGHT BLONDE
9	VERY LIGHT BLONDE
10	LIGHTEST BLONDE

Achieving natural hair colors with the Level System. *(Photographs courtesy of Eric Von Lockhart, top; and Steven Landis, middle and bottom.)*

Plate 20. The Level System. *(Guideline to determine natural hair color. © 1990 Clairol Inc. Reprinted courtesy of Clairol Inc.)*

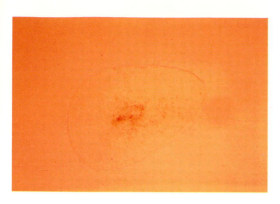

Plate 21

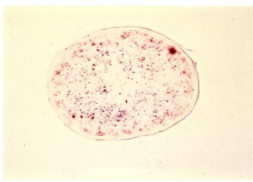

Plate 22

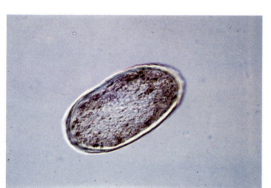

Plate 23

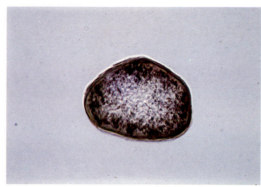

Plate 24

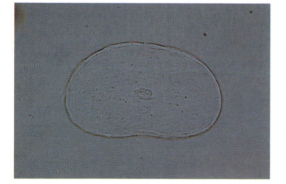

Plate 25

Plate 26

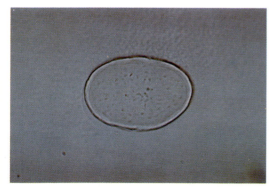

Plate 27

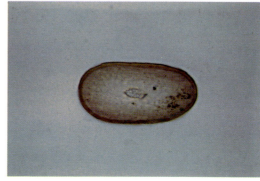

Plate 28

Plate 21. Virgin blonde hair in a henna solution. *(Courtesy: Redken Laboratories, Inc.)*

Plate 22. Cross-section of hair strand saturated with henna for 12 hours. *(Courtesy: Redken Laboratories, Inc.)*

Plate 23. Dark molecules are artificial pigment molecules deposited in permanent tinting. *(Courtesy: Redken Laboratories, Inc.)*

Plate 24. The greater number of molecules in this picture indicated a darker color was achieved. *(Courtesy: Redken Laboratories, Inc.)*

Plate 25. This cross-section view of the hair shaft shows that virgin white hair contains few melanin molecules to absorb light rays. *(Courtesy: Redken Laboratories, Inc.)*

Plate 26. This cross-section of the hair shaft shows albino hair after tinting. This type of hair has no melanin base to which artificial color could attach itself. *(Courtesy: Redken Laboratories, Inc.)*

Plate 27. Virgin white hair has minute melanin molecules, therefore some tint is able to attach. *(Courtesy: Redken Laboratories, Inc.)*

Plate 28. Gray hair generally contains sufficient melanin to allow good color attachment. *(Courtesy: Redken Laboratories, Inc.)*

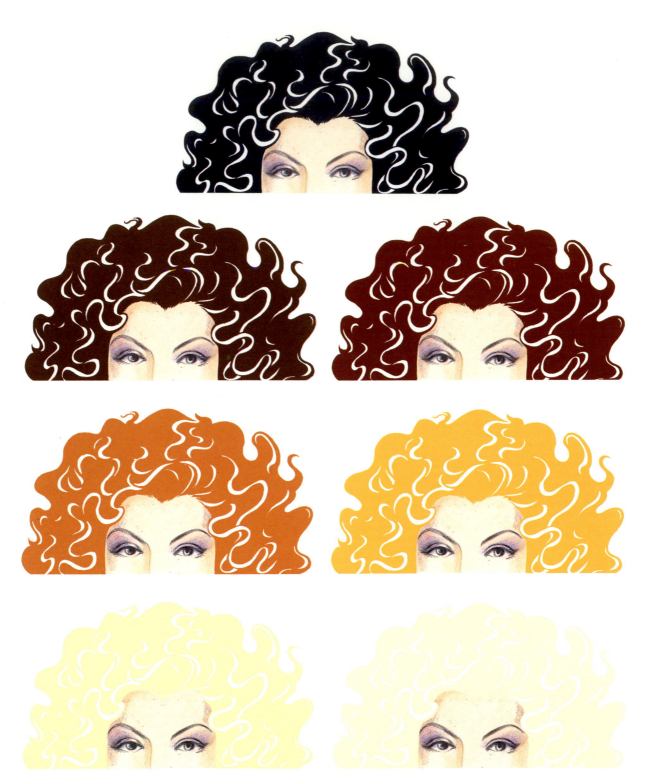

Plate 29. The Seven Stages of Hair Lightening

6
Fillers

A filler is a dual purpose hair coloring product. Fillers have the ability to create a color base and equalize excessive porosity caused by heat, chemical treatments, or exposure to the elements. Simply put, fillers can even porosity while doing color correction. Fillers fall into two general classifications: *protein* and *nonprotein*. Within these two classifications fillers are manufactured in gel, cream, and liquid form, and in a variety of colors as well as clear and neutral.

CHEMICAL AND PHYSICAL ACTION OF FILLERS

Fillers are absorbed by the hair shaft on the basis of porosity. The greater the porosity, the greater the absorption of filler. Inside the cortex, the filler molecules fill in the spaces left in the shaft from prior diffusion of melanin. This creates a base to which tint molecules can now attach.

As the filler penetrates into the cortex, some of the pigment is trapped in the "holes" left by missing cuticle, creating a smooth and even surface on the shaft. This allows for the reflection of more light, which the eye in turn interprets as warmth and sheen. Through this process fillers help to prevent the flat, dull color that can result when tinting damaged hair.

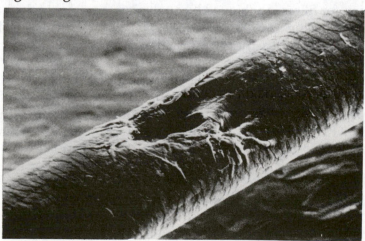

"Holes" in the hair shaft, such as this one caused by chlorine bleach, may be treated with fillers to create more even and longer lasting color.   (Courtesy: Redken Laboratories, Inc.)

Generally the ends of the shaft are more faded and porous than the hair at the scalp. Filler "grabs" more in the porous ends and creates a more consistent shaft from scalp to ends. Both the filling in of the excessive porosity of the cuticle and creation of a color base in the cortex improve the hair's ability to hold color and resist premature removal through shampooing and exposure to the elements.

The action of a filler also prevents color streaking. Sometimes the unevenness of porosity is scattered through the head instead of being uniformly more porous toward the ends of the shaft. This occurs especially when coloring over a prior weaving, highlighting, painting, or frosting. The use of a filler will help to even the porosity and color base throughout the hair, allowing the tint to process without streaking.

Fillers are often used during a tint back to natural. The ability to fill and even porosity and achieve color correction creates an enriched color base that provides improved control of the color results.

COLOR SELECTION

Fillers are available in clear, neutral, and a wide variety of colors as well. The clear filler equalizes porosity but deposits no color base. A clear filler is designed to be used when porosity needs correcting, but color does not.

A neutral filler is a balance of all three primary colors to create a neutral color base. The level of depth is very high (approximately a level 10) and the saturation minimal. A neutral filler does very little color correction but has full power to equalize porosity.

The colored fillers are pre-oxidized color. This means that "What you see is what you get!" To test the hue, depth, and saturation of a filler before use, follow these two steps:

1. Shake the bottle well.
2. Pour a small amount of filler onto a white paper towel or piece of cotton.

After determining the three dimensions of color, neutral, clear, and colored fillers can be mixed together in varying amounts utilizing the Artist's Concept of The Laws of Color to warm, cool, intensify, desaturate, darken, or lighten a filler.

Color selection for fillers is achieved by analyzing the color of the hair to determine the missing hue. By using the Artist's Concept of The Laws of Color, the colorist can add the missing colors to the formula, thereby correcting the color before the problem occurs in tinting.

For example, a common problem that occurs with a tint back to natural on bleached hair is that the hair turns green. Knowing that yellow (the color of bleached hair) and green (the predominant base color of brown tints) create olive (not a great color for hair), the colorist can correct the problem before it occurs by filling the hair with a neutralizing tone of red-orange before or during the tint application.

In addition to correcting any unwanted tone either before or after it is achieved, fillers can be used to enhance a tone. For example, it is common for red tints to fade to orange. This is easily corrected by adding red filler to the tint formula or to the hair shaft prior to tinting.

When formulating, it is important to remember that a filler is milder than a tint and therefore will be somewhat overpowered by it. When first working with fillers, most colorists are surprised at the apparent intensity of the filler color when it is first applied and do not realize that it will be subdued by the tint. Experimentation with hair swatches in all the methods of filler use is recommended to gain a complete background in their use before working on clients.

CHEMICAL COMPOSITION OF PROTEIN FILLERS

Protein fillers are made from inexpensive waste protein materials such as turkey feathers, scrap leather, and hooves of cattle. To prepare the protein, it is ground and pressure cooked with a caustic soda. It then becomes a hydrolysate, or hydrolyzed protein. The proteins treated in this manner are broken down into peptides known as peptones, proteoses, and free-amino acids.

These small chains of polypeptides, soluble in water, are similar to the short chain polypeptides that are created with porosity and protrude from the ends of the hair shaft (unless the hair is so damaged that they have been washed away). Both the damaged hair and the hydrolyzed protein contain freed positive and negative atoms. When they come in contact with each other, the positively charged chains attract the negatively charged chains. In this manner the hair and the protein form salt bonds between each other, attaching the protein to the hair.

The addition of hydrochloric acid or sulfuric acid brings the pH of the mixture within the neutral range of 7.0-7.5. hydrochloric acid, doubling as a solvent, is a clear colorless corrosive liquid that is also used in hair bleaches. Sulfuric acid, with a trade name of "Oil of Vitrol," is a clear, colorless, odorless oily acid that is also used to stimulate appetite.

Cationic compounds work in conjunction with the protein content of fillers to even out the porosity and increase spreadability of the product. Cationic compounds are positively charged and thus attract the negative charges of damaged hair.

Some protein fillers also contain lanolin and cholesterol to protect hair against the harshness of further chemical treatments. Lanolin is a product of the oil glands of sheep. Chemically it is a wax, not a fat, as generally believed. It absorbs and holds water to the hair and prevents excessive drying. Cholesterol is a fat-soluble, crystalline, steroid alcohol that occurs in all animal fats and oils, blood, nervous tissue, and egg yolk. It works as a lubricant and emulsifier.

Fillers use a wide variety of certified color pigments as colorants. This means that the pigments have been certified by the Food and Drug Administration as "harmless and suitable for use."

CHEMICAL COMPOSITION OF NONPROTEIN FILLERS

A few clear gel fillers are not protein fillers. They are made from oil and water emulsions that are thickened or gelled with a mildly acid pH of approximately 3.5-4.0. These fillers are mixtures of the same oils and fatty acids as protein fillers, but use cationic compounds solely as their active ingredient rather than including a protein to cause the product to adhere to the shaft.

SAFETY

Fillers are extremely safe products. The certified coloring pigments used in fillers are known to cause no allergic reaction; thus no predisposition test is needed. The only ingredient in fillers that is known to cause allergy problems is lanolin. However, currently most manufacturers use a derivative of lanolin that is not guilty of causing reaction.

Inhalation or ingestion of an undiluted solution of hydrochloric or sulfuric acid can be hazardous to the health, but as packaged for use by the color industry, it is considered safe.

Use of Gloves

Fillers are nonallergenic, nontoxic, and non-caustic. Therefore, the use of gloves is not required. However, all the characteristics that make fillers adhere so well to the hair cause them to adhere equally well to the skin. To avoid unsightly color stains on the hands, gloves are recommended.

APPLICATION METHODS

Application Method #1—Creates a minimal amount of filling and color correction.

1. Add up to 1 ounce of the desired filler into the tint formulation.
2. Apply tint as usual.

Application Method #2—Creates a moderate amount of filling and color correction.

1. Shampoo and towel dry hair.
2. Apply desired filler to hair.
3. Allow to process for 5-45 minutes.
4. When desired filling is achieved, rinse thoroughly and either towel dry or place client under cool dryer to dry hair completely. To avoid irritation to the scalp, do not blow dry.
5. Apply tint as usual.

Application Method #3—Creates a maximum amount of filling and color correction.

1. Shampoo and towel dry hair.
2. Apply desired filler to hair.
3. Place client under cool dryer and dry filler into hair.
4. Apply tint on top of filler in the usual manner.

If analysis of the hair indicates that the color is balanced and no tones are missing, then either a clear, a neutral, or a filler of the same color as the hair can be used to treat only the porosity of the shaft. Select the method of application from above based on the amount of porosity correction necessary.

CONDITIONER MIXED WITH FILLERS

Fillers are often successfully used in conjunction with conditioning to solve discoloration problems. This formula achieves the very mildest form of filling and is desirable when only a slight amount of color correction or porosity control is necessary. Such instances might be to darken the lightening effects that permanent waving has on some hair, to correct the effects of sun, wind, salt, or chlorinated water, or to blend tinted hair that has faded.

The white cream conditioners are most popular for mixing with fillers. However, polymer based conditioners are the exception. The chemical reaction between these two products may create a white film on the hair that can flake and peel.

Formulation of Filler with Conditioner

1. Place ½ ounce desired filler or mixture of filler colors in nonmetallic mixing receptacle.
2. Add ½ ounce of white cream conditioner (nonpolymer).
3. Stir to blend thoroughly.

Application

1. Shampoo and towel dry hair.
2. Apply to areas needing color correction with a color applicator brush.
3. Processing time varies widely. Five to forty-five minutes may be required to achieve desired color correction.
4. Work into rest of hair to break the line of demarcation.
5. When desired color is achieved, rinse thoroughly and style.

FILLER COLOR CHART

Color selection with fillers is relatively simple. "What you see is what you get!" For this reason, most manufacturers do not make a color chart for their filler line. They assume the colorist can just sample the filler color on a white cotton ball when formulating. However, repeatedly done, this can be a waste of the colorist's time and product.

Objectives

To create a chart of filler colors that will serve as a ready reference for selection and formulation.

Directions

Apply filler on a small cotton ball. Work through and spread the cotton so that the color is apparent. Glue the cotton balls in the spaces indicated and write in the color name and number in the space provided.

#1 _____ #2 _____ #3 _____ #4 _____

#5 _____ #6 _____ #7 _____ #8 _____

#9 _____ #10 _____ #11 _____ #12 _____

WHITE AND SILVER TONING WITH FILLERS
COLOR CORRECTION ON HAIR INSUFFICIENTLY LIGHTENED
EXPERIMENT INSTRUCTION SHEET

Objectives

To observe and document the action of fillers used in conjunction with white and silver toners when a maximum of color correction and porosity control are desired.

Hair Swatches Needed

4 hair swatches bleached to yellow (lighten)

Labeling Hair Swatches

Label swatches as follows:

- White toner with filler
- White toner without filler
- Silver toner with filler
- Silver toner without filler

Materials Needed

- 20 volume hydrogen peroxide
- Violet filler
- Silver permanent toner
- White permanent toner
- Nonmetallic mixing receptacles

Formulation and Application of Filler

1. Place 1 teaspoon of violet filler in a nonmetallic mixing receptacle.
2. Place the strands *labeled for filler application* in filler and swish around until thoroughly saturated.
3. Place under dryer until completely dry.

Formulation and Application of Toners

1. Place 1 teaspoon of each toner in separate nonmetallic mixing receptacles.
2. Add 20 volume hydrogen peroxide and stir.

3. Apply white toner to one swatch with filler and one swatch without filler.
4. Apply silver toner to one swatch with filler and one swatch without filler.
5. Process at room temperature for 35 minutes.
6. Rinse with cool water, shampoo, and dry.
7. Mount swatches on the *Experiment Results Sheet on page R-81.*
8. Answer *Review Questions on page R-83.*

BLONDE TINTING WITH FILLERS

EXPERIMENT INSTRUCTION SHEET

Objectives

To observe and document the action of fillers used in conjunction with blonde tints when a moderate amount of color correction and porosity control is desired.

Hair Swatches Needed

6 damaged hair swatches:

- Level 8-9—Blonde hair

Labeling Hair Swatches

Label swatches as follows:

- Warm blonde tint with filler
- Warm blonde tint without filler
- Neutral blonde tint with filler
- Neutral blonde tint without filler
- Ash blonde tint with filler
- Ash blonde tint without filler

Materials Needed

- Three level 6-7 blonde tints of different bases—warm, neutral, and ash
- 20 volume hydrogen peroxide
- Yellow filler
- Neutral filler
- Violet filler
- Nonmetallic mixing receptacles

Formulation and Application of Fillers

1. Place 1 teaspoon of each filler in a nonmetallic mixing receptacle.
2. Place the swatch labeled "warm blonde with filler" in the yellow based filler.
3. Place the swatch labeled "neutral blonde with filler" in the neutral filler.
4. Place the swatch labeled "ash blonde with filler" in the violet based filler.
5. Swish all swatches around in their containers to insure thorough saturation.
6. Process at room temperature for 30 minutes.
7. Rinse thoroughly and towel dry.

Formulation and Application of Blonde Tints

1. Place 1 teaspoon of each tint in separate mixing receptacles.
2. Add 20 volume hydrogen peroxide according to the manufacturer's recommended directions and stir.
3. Apply the warm tint to the two swatches labeled "warm blonde with/without filler."
4. Apply the neutral tint to the two swatches labeled "neutral blonde with/without filler."
5. Apply the ash tint to the two swatches labeled "ash blonde with/without filler."
6. Process at room temperature for 35 minutes.
7. Rinse with cool water, shampoo, and dry.
8. Mount swatches on the *Experiment Results Sheet on page R-85*.
9. Answer *Review Questions on page R-87*.

BROWN TINTING WITH FILLERS

EXPERIMENT INSTRUCTION SHEET

Objectives

To observe and document the action of fillers used in conjunction with brown tints when a minimal amount of color correction and porosity control are desired.

Hair Swatches Needed

6 damaged hair swatches

Labeling Hair Swatches

Label swatches as follows:

- Light brown tint with filler
- Light brown tint without filler
- Medium brown tint with filler

- Medium brown tint without filler
- Dark brown tint with filler
- Dark brown tint without filler

Materials Needed

- 20 volume H_2O_2
- Level 2—Dark brown tint
- Level 3—Medium brown tint
- Level 4—Light brown tint
- Orange filler
- Red filler
- 6 nonmetallic receptacles

Formulation and Application

1. In the first nonmetallic receptacle mix:

   - 1 teaspoon of light brown tint
   - H_2O_2 according to manufacturer's recommended directions

2. In the second nonmetallic receptacle mix:

   - 1 teaspoon of light brown tint
   - H_2O_2 according to manufacturer's recommended directions
   - 1 teaspoon of orange based filler

3. In the third nonmetallic receptacle mix:

   - 1 teaspoon of light brown tint
   - H_2O_2 according to manufacturer's recommended directions

4. In the fourth nonmetallic receptacle mix:

   - 1 teaspoon of medium brown tint
   - H_2O_2 according to manufacturer's recommended directions
   - 1 teaspoon of orange based filler

5. In the fifth nonmetallic receptacle mix:

   - 1 teaspoon of dark brown tint
   - H_2O_2 according to manufacturer's recommended directions

6. In the sixth nonmetallic receptacle mix:

   - 1 teaspoon of dark brown tint
   - H_2O_2 according to manufacturer's recommended directions
   - 1 teaspoon of red based filler

7. Apply each formulation to the appropriately marked swatch.
8. Process at room temperature for 35 minutes.
9. Rinse with cool water, shampoo, and dry.
10. Mount swatches on the *Experiment Results Sheet on page R-89.*
11. Answer *Review Questions on page R-91.*

REFRESHING TINTED RED HAIR WITH FILLERS

EXPERIMENT INSTRUCTION SHEET

Objectives

To observe and document the action of fillers used in conjunction with conditioners to refresh red shades of tinted hair.

Hair Swatches Needed

3 tinted hair swatches of the following color levels:

- Level 6-7—Light red
- Level 4-5—Medium red
- Level 3—Burgundy red

Labeling Hair Swatches

Label the 3 swatches according to their level

Materials Needed

- Red filler
- Violet filler
- Gold filler
- 3 nonmetallic mixing receptacles
- Plastic wrap

Formulation and Application

1. Mix ½ teaspoon gold filler, ½ teaspoon red filler, and 1 teaspoon of conditioner in first receptacle.
2. Mix 1 teaspoon red filler and 1 teaspoon conditioner in second receptacle.
3. Mix ½ teaspoon of red filler, ½ teaspoon of violet filler, and 1 teaspoon conditioner in third receptacle

Procedure

1. Apply the first formula to the freshly shampooed level 6-7 light red swatch.
2. Apply the second formula to the freshly shampooed level 4-5 medium red swatch.
3. Apply the third formula to the freshly shampooed level 3 burgundy swatch.
4. Wrap swatches individually in plastic.
5. Process in a warm dryer for 5 minutes.
6. Strand test every 5 minutes until the color is refreshed.
7. Rinse thoroughly (do not shampoo) and dry swatches.
8. Mount swatches on the *Experiment Results Sheet on page R-93.*
9. Answer *Review Questions on page R-95.*

7

Reds, Reds, and More Reds

Redheads are vivacious, outgoing, unpredictable, and slightly hot tempered. Dealing with a redhead is much like working with the color red. If you do not take the time to understand it, you may find yourself wishing you had!

Most shades of hair have a sulfur content of 4-5 percent. Natural red hair contains up to 8 percent. Thus natural red hair may contain twice as many sulfur bonds as all other shades. This high sulfur content makes the hair more resistant and difficult to treat chemically.

HISTORY

Red hair also has problems with fashion stability. It seems to be a color that is either loved or hated. Red as a hair color has swayed violently from one side of the pendulum to the other.

In early times antipathy for red hair stemmed from the belief that Judas, betrayer of Christ, was a redhead. The saying "Judas colored hair" was popular in many languages. This repugnance to red hair was reinforced by the theory that Cain, the first recorded murderer, had red hair. The fat of a dead redhead was ever in demand as an ingredient in poison.

In England and the north of France, this common dislike of red hair was kept alive by the repeated invasions of the Danes, a red-haired race. However, the Danes themselves considered their red hair to be a sign of strength.

European opinion during the 1500's ran from a mild distrust of redheads to a belief that all red-haired women were witches. Many were hunted down and tortured and killed because of the color of their hair.

Red hair enjoyed a time of fashion popularity during the 1600's with the coronation of Elizabeth, a natural redhead, as the Queen of England. The ladies of Queen Elizabeth's court dyed their hair or wore red wigs in efforts to emulate their revered queen. When it was decreed legal for common women to redden their hair for the purpose of giving their husbands pleasure, ladies openly experimented with home concoctions to achieve this new fashion look.

In 16th century Italy, red hair was given the name *imbalconata* from the custom of displaying red rose bushes. Bushes in full bloom were arranged on the balcony to impress the neighbors with the beautiful flowers.

Lucille Ball was probably the most popular redhead of all time. The vivaciousness and unpredictability of her character on the "I Love Lucy Show" became personality traits attributed to redheads yet today. However, it must be noted that Sarah Ferguson ("Fergie") certainly gave red hair a boost in popularity after the royal wedding in July of 1986.

Whatever traits attributed to the color red, it is never stagnant or boring. Studies indicate that more red cars than any other color are involved in automobile accidents as well as receive more speeding tickets. Red is known to cause anger in many animals. Particularly famous cases are the charging bull and the biting bee.

Red historically causes problems for the hair colorist as well. Red, more than any other tinted shade, has the tendency to turn excessively brassy, fade easily, and process off-color to violet or pink. Red is the most difficult color to match because of its vibrancy and highly reflective qualities.

Red is also the most difficult color for a client to communicate to the colorist. Most clients asking to be "redheads" really want to be "orangeheads"!

UNWANTED BRASSINESS

Unwanted brassiness has plagued redheads for centuries. Marie Eugenie de Montijo, wife of Napoleon III and empress of France, considered her own red shade to be too harsh. Therefore, she dusted her hair with a fine gold powder to soften its brassiness.

Excessive brassiness occurs more frequently in tinting the hair to red than any other hue. The ammonia in permanent tints tends to bring out red, orange, and yellow in the natural hair color. This underlying red added to the red dye can lead to more warmth than expected.

FADEAGE

Fading is a common problem of tinted red hair. The combination of ammonia and peroxide in the tinting formula diffuses the natural pigment within the hair shaft resulting in the smaller melanin molecules within the shaft. The artificial pigments attach to the diffused melanin to create a new hue of hair color. However, with every subsequent shampooing, blow-drying, permanent waving, sun exposure, or dousing in salt or chlorinated water, the artificial pigment is removed through the porosity of the cuticle. The greater the porosity, the quicker the color fades. This loosening of the attached color pigments leaves behind the smaller diffused melanin molecules, which now are of the structure to reflect light rays within the red, orange, and yellow range. This warmth caused by the oxidation process can be considered excessive.

PREVENTING BRASSINESS

As the artificial pigment fades and the brassiness becomes apparent, the natural tendency of the client is to request more frequent retouches. Rescheduling retouches at closer and closer intervals causes greater porosity and diffusion of the natural pigment, leaving the hair brassier than ever before as the tint once again fades. A never-ending cycle begins.

The first step to devising a solution to this situation is to determine the cause of the fading. If the client is a sun-worshiper the color may fade from week to week. A scarf or hat provides protection from the sun's oxidizing ultra violet rays. The use of hair care products containing ultra violet absorbers can help to provide a protective barrier between the shaft and the sun. Long haired clients can saturate their hair with conditioner and wear it braided or twisted into a chignon to protect their tinted tresses.

At least rinsing, preferably shampooing and conditioning, salt and chlorinated water from the hair immediately after emerging will lessen the damaging effects on the hair. The application of less heat of any form to the hair will also help to prevent damage to the cuticle and diffusion of artificial and natural color molecules. Also, a milder permanent waving solution should be advised for those clients who do combine color and perming.

Protein treatments will help to fill in the porosity of the hair and protect it from the elements and artificial abuse. However, strong protein treatments (the brown liquid type) should be given the week before the tinting service rather than immediately after, because the protein does open cuticle somewhat as it attaches itself to the hair shaft and this can cause a fresh tint to fade.

Use of a lower volume of hydrogen peroxide can also prevent excessive brassiness. If the desired depth of red is of the same or deeper level than the natural color, the hue can be achieved through deposition without excessive lift. The lower volume of peroxide will reduce the amount of diffusion of melanin and thus the reflection of red, orange, and yellow wavelengths. This technique can be particularly useful in achieving and retaining the violet based reds.

CORRECTING EXCESSIVE BRASSINESS

The first step to camouflage excessive brassiness in either natural or tinted hair is to analyze it. Is it red, yellow, or orange? Then refer to the Chromatic Circle. Locate the particular shade of brassiness and draw a line directly across on the circle to find the hue that will neutralize the unwanted shade.

Now that the neutralizing hue is identified, a number of options exist for solving the problem.

Solution #1—Temporary Rinses

Select two temporary rinses, one that is as close as possible to the red shade desired and one that has the same base color as the corresponding neutralizing hue on the Chromatic Circle. Mix a small amount with one part red and one part of the neutralizing hue. If the color is still too brassy, increase the amount of the neutralizing hue. If the color is over-neutralized and becomes too cool, then increase the amount of red rinse.

This method can be used on tinted hair in between retouches or on virgin hair to neutralize brassiness.

Solution #2—Neutralizing Tint Formulas

Brassiness can be neutralized during the soap cap stage of a retouch. Add a small amount of tint with a neutralizing hue (no additional peroxide) to the soap cap. Perform a test strand for formulation correctness.

This method is for tinted hair only, unless the client is ready to commit to monthly coloring services.

Solution #3—Fillers

Any of the standard application methods of fillers can effectively cut brassiness by mixing the hue of filler that will neutralize the excessive warmth as matched on the color wheel.

This method is effective only on tinted red hair. Fillers attach to the hair shaft on the basis of porosity or deposition with the aid of a penetrating product. Therefore, they generally do not give satisfactory color correction used alone on virgin hair.

Solution #4—Semipermanent Colors

Semipermanent colors of a neutralizing shade can be effective in neutralizing brass in virgin hair. Because most permanent tints and semipermanent rinses are not compatible, this method is not generally used on tinted hair. Check the directions on the individual semipermanent rinse to see if the manufacturer states that it is compatible with tint. If not, use an alternate method.

RED TINTING ON NATURAL LEVEL 2—DARK BROWN

EXPERIMENT INSTRUCTION SHEET

Objectives

To observe and document the color results when tinting to red on level 2—Dark brown hair.

Hair Swatches Needed

4 virgin hair swatches—Level 2—Dark brown

Labeling Hair Swatches

Label Swatches as follows:

- Level 9—Name of the red tint you selected for use
- Level 7—Name of the red tint you selected for use
- Level 5—Name of the red tint you selected for use
- Level 3—Name of the red tint you selected for use

Materials Needed

- 20 volume hydrogen peroxide
- Four red tints: Level 9, Level 7, Level 5, and Level 3
- Nonmetallic mixing receptacles

Procedure

1. Mix 1 teaspoon of each tint with the appropriate amount of hydrogen peroxide in nonmetallic mixing receptacles.
2. Process at room temperature for 40 minutes.
3. Rinse with cool water, shampoo, and dry.
4. Mount swatches on the *Experiment Results Sheet on page R-97.*
5. Answer *Review Questions on page R-99.*

RED TINTING ON NATURAL LEVEL 5—LIGHTEST BROWN

EXPERIMENT INSTRUCTION SHEET

Objectives

To observe and document the color results when tinting to red on level 5—Lightest brown hair.

Hair Swatches Needed

4 virgin hair swatches—Level 5—Lightest brown

Labeling Hair Swatches

- Level 9—Name of the red tint you selected for use
- Level 7—Name of the red tint you selected for use
- Level 5—Name of the red tint you selected for use
- Level 3—Name of the red tint you selected for use

Materials Needed

- 20 volume hydrogen peroxide
- Four red tints: Level 9, Level 7, Level 5, and Level 3
- Nonmetallic mixing receptacles

Procedure

1. Mix 1 teaspoon of each tint with the appropriate amount of hydrogen peroxide in nonmetallic mixing receptacles.
2. Process at room temperature for 40 minutes.
3. Rinse with cool water, shampoo, and dry.
4. Mount swatches on the *Experiment Results Sheet on page R-101.*
5. Answer *Review Questions on page R-103.*

RED TINTING ON NATURAL LEVEL 8—LIGHT BLONDE

EXPERIMENT INSTRUCTION SHEET

Objectives

To observe and document the color results when tinting to red on level 8—Light blonde hair.

Hair Swatches Needed

4 virgin hair swatches—Level 8—Light blonde

Labeling Hair Swatches

- Level 9—Name of the red tint you selected for use
- Level 7—Name of the red tint you selected for use
- Level 5—Name of the red tint you selected for use
- Level 3—Name of the red tint you selected for use

Materials Needed

- 20 volume hydrogen peroxide
- Four red tints: Level 9, Level 7, Level 5, and Level 3
- Nonmetallic mixing receptacles

Procedure

1. Mix 1 teaspoon of each tint with the appropriate amount of hydrogen peroxide in nonmetallic mixing receptacles.
2. Process at room temperature for 40 minutes.
3. Rinse with cool water, shampoo, and dry.
4. Mount swatches on the *Experiment Results Sheet on page R-105.*
5. Answer *Review Questions on page R-107.*

8

Tint Back to Natural Color

Many reasons exist for clients to want or need a tint back to natural. Often clients who have been either tinting or bleaching will want to return to their natural shade. Sun, chlorinated swimming pool water, or prior chemical services can alter the hair color. In all of these cases, the process is too complex to be successfully performed by the average consumer. Therefore, the tint back to natural can be an excellent source of income for the professional colorist.

Several factors make a tint back to natural the most complex of the basic color applications. Formulation to match the natural color on hair that has received many previous coloring treatments requires a complete understanding of the Laws of Color. The unevenness of porosity from scalp to ends requires that the timing of this process must be adjusted to achieve even color. This type of hair may absorb color very quickly and process darker and cooler than expected. The natural pigment may be so diffused that it will not accept the color at all. And as if these factors did not complicate things enough, this hair tends to fade faster than normal.

The solution to a successful tint back to natural can lie in the use of a filler to even out the porosity and achieve color correction. Refer to the section on fillers for the three standard methods of use to decide which is appropriate for the amount of porosity in each individual situation.

Formulations incorporating the theories of low volume peroxide are often used for a tint back to natural. This milder solution that does no lifting as it deposits is less damaging.

To avoid the ash tones that characteristically appear when tinting over-porous hair, refer to the color wheel. Use the artist's theory of neutralization of unwanted tones in formulating to create the warmth necessary to prevent a drab, unnatural looking color in the finished product.

Performing a test strand is a *must* when preparing to do a tint back to natural. The condition of the hair, the change in texture, the reduced moisture content and elasticity, the increase and unevenness of the porosity, set the stage for unpredictable color results. Each case is different!

117

TINT BACK TO NATURAL LEVEL 6—DARK BLONDE ON BLEACHED HAIR

EXPERIMENT INSTRUCTION SHEET

Objectives

To observe and document the color results of a tint back to a natural level 6—Dark blonde on bleached hair using different formulations. To gain experience formulating and mixing product, implementing concepts of varying volumes of hydrogen peroxide, use of additives, and the Laws of Color.

Hair Swatches Needed

6 bleached blonde hair swatches

Labeling Hair Swatches

Label swatches as follows:

- 20 volume H_2O_2 and ash blonde
- 20 volume H_2O_2 and warm blonde
- 10 volume H_2O_2 and ash blonde
- 10 volume H_2O_2 and warm blonde
- 20 volume H_2O_2, filler, and ash blonde
- 20 volume H_2O_2, filler, and warm blonde

Materials Needed

- 20 volume H_2O_2
- 10 volume H_2O_2
- Yellow based filler
- Level 6—Dark warm blonde tint
- Level 6—Dark ash blonde tint
- 6 nonmetallic mixing receptacles

Formulation

1. *Swatch #1*—Mix 1 teaspoon of ash blonde tint with appropriate amount of 20 volume hydrogen peroxide in nonmetallic mixing receptacle.
2. *Swatch #2*—Mix 1 teaspoon of warm blonde tint with appropriate amount of 20 volume hydrogen peroxide in nonmetallic mixing receptacle.
3. *Swatch #3*—Mix 1 teaspoon of ash blonde tint with appropriate amount of 10 volume hydrogen peroxide in nonmetallic mixing receptacle.

4. *Swatch #4*—Mix 1 teaspoon of warm blonde tint with appropriate amount of 10 volume hydrogen peroxide in nonmetallic mixing receptacle.
5. *Swatch #5*—Mix ½ teaspoon of ash blonde tint with appropriate amount of 20 volume hydrogen peroxide and add ½ teaspoon of yellow based filler in nonmetallic mixing receptacle.
6. *Swatch #6*—Mix ½ teaspoon of warm blonde tint with appropriate amount of 20 volume hydrogen peroxide and add ½ teaspoon of yellow based filler in nonmetallic mixing receptacle.

Procedure

1. Apply each formulation to the appropriately marked swatch.
2. Process at room temperature for 35 minutes.
3. Rinse with cool water, shampoo, and dry.
4. Mount swatches on the *Experiment Results Sheet on page R-109.*
5. Answer *Review Questions on page R-111.*

TINT BACK TO NATURAL LEVEL 4—MEDIUM BROWN ON BLEACHED HAIR

EXPERIMENT INSTRUCTION SHEET

Objectives

To observe and document the color results on a tint back to a natural level 4—Medium brown on bleached hair using different formulations. To gain experience formulating and mixing product, implementing concepts of varying volumes of hydrogen peroxide, use of additives, and the Laws of Color.

Hair Swatches Needed

6 bleached blonde hair swatches

Labeling Hair Swatches

Label swatches as follows:

- 20 volume H_2O_2 and ash brown
- 20 volume H_2O_2 and warm brown
- 10 volume H_2O_2 and ash brown
- 10 volume H_2O_2 and warm brown
- 20 volume H_2O_2, filler, and ash brown
- 20 volume H_2O_2, filler, and warm brown

Materials Needed

- 20 volume H_2O_2
- 10 volume H_2O_2
- Orange based filler
- Level 4—Medium ash brown tint
- Level 4—Medium warm brown tint
- 6 nonmetallic mixing receptacles

Formulation

1. *Swatch #1*—Mix 1 teaspoon of ash brown tint with appropriate amount of 20 volume hydrogen peroxide in nonmetallic mixing receptacle.
2. *Swatch #2*—Mix 1 teaspoon of warm brown tint with appropriate amount of 20 volume hydrogen peroxide in nonmetallic mixing receptacle.
3. *Swatch #3*—Mix 1 teaspoon of ash brown tint with appropriate amount of 10 volume hydrogen peroxide in nonmetallic mixing receptacle.
4. *Swatch #4*—Mix 1 teaspoon of warm brown tint with appropriate amount of 10 volume hydrogen peroxide in nonmetallic mixing receptacle.
5. *Swatch #5*—Mix ½ teaspoon of ash brown tint with appropriate amount of 20 volume hydrogen peroxide and add ½ teaspoon of orange based filler in nonmetallic mixing receptacle.
6. *Swatch #6*—Mix ½ teaspoon of warm brown tint with appropriate amount of 20 volume hydrogen peroxide and add ½ teaspoon of orange based filler in nonmetallic mixing receptacle.

Procedure

1. Process at room temperature for 35 minutes.
2. Rinse with cool water, shampoo, and dry.
3. Mount swatches on the *Experiment Results Sheet on page R-113.*
5. Answer *Review Questions on page R-115.*

TINT BACK TO NATURAL LEVEL 2—DARK BROWN ON BLEACHED HAIR

EXPERIMENT INSTRUCTION SHEET

Objectives

To observe and document the color results of a tint back to a natural level 2—Dark brown on bleached hair using three different formulations. To gain experience formulating and mixing product, implementing concepts of varying volumes of hydrogen peroxide, use of additives, and the Laws of Color.

Hair Swatches Needed

6 bleached blonde hair swatches

Labeling Hair Swatches

Label swatches as follows:

- 20 volume H_2O_2 and dark ash brown
- 20 volume H_2O_2 and dark warm brown
- 10 volume H_2O_2 and dark ash brown
- 10 volume H_2O_2 and dark warm brown
- 20 volume H_2O_2, filler, and dark ash brown
- 20 volume H_2O_2, filler, and dark warm brown

Materials Needed

- 20 volume H_2O_2
- 10 volume H_2O_2
- Red based filler
- Level 2—Dark warm brown tint
- Level 2—Dark ash brown tint
- 6 nonmetallic mixing receptacles

Formulation

1. *Swatch #1*—Mix 1 teaspoon of dark ash brown tint with appropriate amount of 20 volume hydrogen peroxide in nonmetallic mixing receptacle.
2. *Swatch #2*—Mix 1 teaspoon of dark warm brown tint with appropriate amount of 20 volume hydrogen peroxide in nonmetallic mixing receptacle.
3. *Swatch #3*—Mix 1 teaspoon of dark ash brown tint with appropriate amount of 10 volume hydrogen peroxide in nonmetallic mixing receptacle.
4. *Swatch #4*—Mix 1 teaspoon of dark warm brown tint with appropriate amount of 10 volume hydrogen peroxide in nonmetallic mixing receptacle.
5. *Swatch #5*—Mix ½ teaspoon of dark ash brown tint with appropriate amount of 20 volume hydrogen peroxide and add ½ teaspoon of red based filler in nonmetallic mixing receptacle.
6. *Swatch #6*—Mix ½ teaspoon of dark warm brown tint with appropriate amount of 20 volume hydrogen peroxide and add ½ teaspoon of red based filler in nonmetallic mixing receptacle.

Procedure

1. Apply each formulation to the appropriately marked swatch.
2. Process at room temperature for 35 minutes.
3. Rinse with cool water, shampoo, and dry.
4. Mount swatches on the *Experiment Results Sheet on page R-117.*
5. Answer *Review Questions on page R-119.*

9
White and Gray Hair

Gray, white, and salt-and-pepper hair have characteristics that create unique coloring problems. A major portion of salon coloring services are performed to either cover or enhance gray. Therefore, this section is dedicated to the study of gray, white, and salt-and-pepper hair, its structure, texture, condition, and in particular the characteristics that make it different from all other colors of hair.

Canities is the technical term for white or gray hair. This condition is divided into two categories according to the age of the person. These two categories are known as *congenital canities* and *acquired canities*.

Congenital canities occurs at or before birth in hair that appears otherwise perfectly normal. It may develop in streaks or patches. It can be solid or blended throughout the head, as in "salt-and-pepper" hair. Albinism, a hereditary condition that falls within this grouping, is a complete lack of pigment in the hair with very little pigment in the skin and eyes.

The classification of acquired canities is further divided into two sub-categories: *normal* and *premature*. Normal graying begins around the age of 35. Even though the loss of pigment progresses in most people through the rest of their lives, few become completely white. Most retain a percentage of pigmented hair.

Generally, premature graying can be traced to hereditary factors. However, it can be brought on by extreme mental, emotional, or physical disorders. Premature graying is occasionally attributed to neuralgia, migraines, anemia, tuberculosis, malaria, or various prolonged illnesses and wasting diseases. It also has been associated with a decreased function of the thyroid and pituitary gland. Traumatic shock has been known to cause normal hair to turn gray within a few hours. Hair may turn gray evenly, in patches, circles, or strips. When the time of shock or stress (whether emotional or physical) has passed, the hair may or may not return to its natural color.

STRUCTURE OF WHITE AND GRAY HAIR

Both gray and white hair contain little melanin within the cortex. Albino and aged white hair basically have no pigment molecules. Because there is no melanin to absorb light rays, all the colors of the visible spectrum are reflected. As discussed earlier in this text, the additive mixing of these wavelengths creates white light; thus the white appearance of this type of hair. *(See Color Plate 25.)*

Hair can appear gray for two different reasons. The first example occurs when the hair contains small amounts of pigment diffused throughout the cortex. This diffused pigment spaced between large air pockets absorbs enough light rays to give the shaft a slight color. The second situation in which the hair appears gray occurs when there is a mixture of white and dark hair. This blending, known as "salt and pepper," creates different shades of gray depending upon the ratio of pigmented to non-pigmented hair.

Gray hair tends to be coarser, less elastic, and occasionally curlier than the other hair on the same head. It also becomes more resistant to chemical services, and thus requires special consideration in hair coloring theory and practicum.

YELLOWED GRAY HAIR

Gray hair can take on a yellow cast for many reasons. Exposure to artificial heat from hair dryers, the elements, and possibly chemicals that oxidize the melanin can create a yellow hue. Yellow tinges may be caused by chlorine, smoking, detergent shampoo, and excessive sebum.

Long hair is particularly susceptible to yellowing. As the hair ages, it is exposed over and over to the instances described above. This creates hair that becomes progressively more yellowed toward the ends. All these factors can cause a stain that sometimes can be removed without harm to the hair by use of a chelator or an oil type color remover.

Yellow may also appear as the body's way of reacting to foods, medicines, or chemicals taken internally. Discoloration created within the cortical layer can be removed only by changing the structure of the hair shaft. Anything taken internally that affects the hair shaft becomes part of the structure of the hair. Removing the yellow from the cortex will remove or destroy parts of the building blocks of the hair structure. Just as removing parts of a block wall will weaken the wall's strength, removing pieces of the building blocks of the hair shaft will weaken it.

Bleach and dye removers will remove yellow discoloration occurring from internal causes or the oxidation of melanin. Undesired yellow can be overpowered by the artificial pigments deposited by tints of an equal or darker level than the yellow. Another option is to neutralize the yellow tones with a comparable level of violet.

CLIENT CONSULTATION

Most non-pigmented hair can be changed to any color classification the client might desire. A head of hair that is a mixture of both pigmented and non-pigmented hair will require more advanced color techniques and theories, but can still be successfully colored. In either case, the colorist should help to guide a client away from the colors that are too dark or too warm.

Many clients initially want to return to the color of their youth. They do not realize that the pigment of their skin is aging in a process similar to that of the hair. The newly produced skin and hair are lighter due to the reduced production of melanin. To tint the hair back to the natural color of their youth creates a severe contrast that can be harsh. Generally, a color of a similar tone but lighter level will be more flattering.

The colorist should consult with the client to determine lifestyle and expectations for this color service. In addition to the color and product selection, the client should be counseled as to cost, maintenance, and time commitment. Gray or white hair is one of the most difficult on which to do a tint back to natural service, so it is recommended that all aspects of this service be thoroughly discussed before a permanent color is applied.

DETERMINING THE PERCENTAGE OF GRAY

Most people retain some dark hair as they turn gray. This hair must be analyzed for level and hue. Successful tinting of gray hair involves one additional step—determining the percentage of gray.

PERCENTAGE OF GRAY	CHARACTERISTICS
100-90%	Virtually no pigmented hair; tends to look white.
90-70%	Mostly non-pigmented hair; generally majority of remaining pigmented hair is located in back with rest blended over head.
70-50%	More gray than pigmented; unnecessary to study hair to see the gray.
50-30%	More pigmented than gray; easy to see in dark colors but may blend in with lighter natural hair.
30-10%	Mostly pigmented; difficult to see; generally most heavily located in temples and sides with some blending of colors throughout head.

COLOR AND PRODUCT SELECTION

The pure white hair of an albino will accept only those hair colorings that are designed to coat the hair. This type of hair has no melanin within the cortical layer of the hair. Therefore, no base or structure exists for the artificial color to affix itself to. Likewise, bleaching is not satisfactory because there is no natural pigment to diffuse and form a foundation for proper toner development. *(See Color Plates 26 and 27.)*

In selecting a coating color, such as a temporary rinse, for application to albino white hair, it is important to remember that the color will not be diluted or affected by the natural color, as it is when the hair is blonde or brown. The rinse will coat the hair and reflect the color of the rinse, just as it comes from the bottle. Therefore, the colorist may have to mix and blend colors to create a balanced shade.

Even though hair that has lightened to white through the ageing process is considered to be non-pigmented, it still contains a small amount of melanin within the cortex. This provides the structure necessary for the artificial pigment of semipermanent and permanent colors to affix themselves. This makes it possible to successfully color gray hair with almost any classification of hair color. *(See Color Plate 28.)*

However, hennas, metallic tints, and semipermanent polymer colors of bright shades generally produce unsatisfactory colors on white or gray hair. The pigment in hennas and vibrant polymers is too concentrated to produce natural looking results on such stark white hair. The metallic tints tend to produce "metallic-looking" shades. Particularly after several uses, the hair may reflect tones of blue, turquoise, or green.

For the most part, however, gray and white hair adapts itself well to the use of any of the three classifications of color. Generally, the selection is dictated by client desires and lifestyle.

TONAL SELECTION

Non-pigmented hair reacts very strongly to the tonal quality of the artificial color whether it is temporary, semipermanent, or permanent. In formulation, varying amounts of all primary pigments must be mixed to achieve a balance of color on white hair.

Gray hair, considered non-pigmented hair, does retain small particles of melanin that reflect light waves that are interpreted by the brain as blue. For that reason, it is generally advised to avoid a blue-based color. The addition of blue pigment to gray hair gives a very drab cast to the hair. A neutral tone used on gray or white hair will achieve a cool tone.

A violet-based color is effective if the gray hair has taken on a yellow cast, but can also give an overly ash color when used on true gray or white hair. This flat gray or muddy appearance that commonly occurs often gives the illusion that the color has not taken or processed properly. To avoid this extreme ash condition, yellow pigment can be added to the formula.

A lack of luster or shine on colored gray or white hair also indicates an over abundance of ash in the resulting color. Warm colors reflect more light than cool colors, making the hair appear shiny. If the color resulting from the test strand appears flat and dull, add a small amount of warmth to the formula.

However, sometimes excessive warmth becomes a problem. When formulating for those clients who are less than 75 to 80 percent gray, the dark hair must be strongly considered because it has a major effect on the tone achieved. The higher the percentage of dark hair on the head, the more red and gold will be seen in the final color when using a lifting tint. Colors that create warm tones on gray or white hair generally will turn the "pepper" hair to brass.

Occasionally this unwanted warmth occurs even when using semipermanent colors. This occurs because of the "self-oxidizing" qualities of the classification of color. An oxidizer has been added to the formula before packaging and although mild, it still can oxidize the natural pigment somewhat and create underlying warmth.

TONAL SELECTION FOR TINTING NON-PIGMENTED HAIR

EXPERIMENT INSTRUCTION SHEET

Objectives

To observe and document the differences and similarities in the tones that can be created by use of one level of tint that is formulated with a variety of base colors.

Hair Swatches Needed

6 non-pigmented hair swatches (either 100 percent or salt and pepper)

Labeling Hair Swatches

Label the hair swatches to indicate the tone of the tint to be applied on each.

- Gold base
- Blue base
- Orange base
- Green base
- Red base
- Violet base

Materials Needed

- 20 volume hydrogen peroxide
- 6 tints of the same level (either level 6—Dark blonde or level 5—Lightest brown) with the varying base colors as indicated above
- Nonmetallic mixing receptacles

Procedure

1. Mix 1 teaspoon of each tint with 20 volume hydrogen peroxide in nonmetallic mixing receptacles.
2. Thoroughly saturate swatches as indicated on labels.
3. Process each swatch at room temperature for 55 minutes. (Remember that standard processing time on non-pigmented hair is 45 minutes. The extra 10 minutes simulates the application time on an entire head.)
4. Shampoo, rinse, and dry each swatch.
5. Mount swatches on the *Experiment Results Sheet on page R-121.*
6. Answer the *Review Questions on page R-123.*

LEVEL SELECTION

Level selection for aged white hair is relatively simple because it accepts basically the level applied. However, colors that are a level 9 or lighter may not give complete coverage because of the small percentage of artificial pigment in these shades. Generally formulations from the levels 6, 7, or 8 will give better coverage and can be used to create pastel and blonde tones if desired.

For those clients who are 80 to 100 percent gray, a hair color within the blonde range is generally more flattering than a darker shade. This lighter level of artificial color may be selected to give a warm or a cool finished product depending upon the client's skin tone, eye color, and personal preferences.

Another factor to be considered when coloring the gray in salt-and-pepper hair to a darker level is that "color on color makes a darker color." The addition of dark artificial pigment to the natural pigment (peppered hair) causes more light rays to be absorbed and less to be reflected. The result is a color that the eye perceives as darker. For this reason, when attempting to cover the gray in a salt-and-pepper head, a shade lighter than the naturally dark hair is generally selected.

A product color chart can be used in conjunction with the following formulation charts to select hues with which to perform a test strand.

SEMIPERMANENT COLOR FORMULATION CHART FOR GRAY HAIR

Percentage of Gray	Formulation
100-90%	Desired level
90-70%	Equal parts desired and lighter level
70-50%	One level lighter
50-30%	Equal parts one level lighter and two levels lighter
30-10%	Two levels lighter

PERMANENT TINT FORMULATION CHART FOR GRAY HAIR

Percentage of Gray	Formulation
100-90%	Desired level
90-70%	Two parts desired level and one part lighter level
70-50%	Equal parts desired and lighter level
50-30%	Two parts lighter level and one part desired level
30-10%	One level lighter

The semipermanent color generally must be selected even lighter than the permanent tint because the semipermanent lacks lifting power. Its ability to only deposit and coat will create a level of color that appears darker than a comparable level in a permanent oxidizing tint.

LEVEL SELECTION FOR TINTING NON-PIGMENTED HAIR

EXPERIMENT INSTRUCTION SHEET

Objectives

To observe and document the differences and similarities in coverage due to level selection. To gain experience in formulating for gray hair coverage.

Hair Swatches Needed

5 non-pigmented hair swatches (either 100 percent or salt and pepper)

Labeling Hair Swatches

Label the hair swatches to indicate the level of tint to be applied on each.

- Level 10—Lightest blonde
- Level 8—Light blonde
- Level 6—Dark blonde
- Level 4—Light brown
- Level 2—Dark brown

Materials Needed

- 20 volume hydrogen peroxide
- 5 tints (same bases) of each level of tint as indicated
- Nonmetallic mixing receptacles

Procedure

1. Mix 1 teaspoon of each tint with 20 volume hydrogen peroxide in nonmetallic mixing receptacle.
2. Thoroughly saturate swatches as indicated on label.
3. Process each strand for 55 minutes. (Remember that standard processing time on non-pigmented hair is 45 minutes. The extra 10 minutes simulates the application time on an entire head.)
4. Shampoo, rinse, and dry each swatch.
5. Mount swatches on the *Experiment Results Sheet on page R-125.*
6. Answer the *Review Questions on page R-127.*

ACHIEVING DESIRED TONE AND LEVEL ON SALT-AND-PEPPER HAIR

Several possible solutions exist to solve problems that occur concerning level and tonality:

1. Pre-lighten the darker hair to artificially create even depth and tonality throughout the head.
2. Formulate a compromise color, one that will not appear too ash on the light hair, yet not create excessive brassiness in the dark hair.
3. Apply a warm tint to the gray hair prior to application of the tint to the entire head.
4. Use two different colors, such as a darker color in the front and a lighter color in the back.

A test strand should be done in both the front and back, on the light and the dark hair, when coloring salt-and-pepper hair. The general rules below can be used to adjust a formula.

Adjusting the Formula Level

To slightly darken a color without changing the tonal value, add small amounts of the color next in depth but of the same base color.

To slightly lighten a color without changing the tonal value, add small amounts of the color next in lightness but of the same base color.

Adjusting the Formula Tone

To cool a color slightly without changing the level, add small amounts of the nearest color on the Chromatic Circle with a cool base (blue, green, violet).

To warm a color slightly without changing the level, add small amounts of the nearest color on the Chromatic Circle with a warm base (yellow, orange, red).

To neutralize an unwanted tone, add the color with the base opposite it on the color wheel.

VOLUME OF HYDROGEN PEROXIDE

Twenty volume hydrogen peroxide is generally recommended when coloring gray hair with permanent tints. The strength created by the combination of ammonia and 20 volume H_2O_2 is necessary to soften and open the cuticle for proper penetration and color development.

Lower volumes of peroxide will usually not open the cuticle sufficiently to allow penetration and cause development of a tint as intended by the manufacturer. A formulation with low volume peroxide may be used to give a slight color change, but it generally fades rapidly as the shallow penetration allows the color to be affected by regular shampooing.

On the other hand, a higher volume of peroxide is not recommended. Gray hair is so light that there is no need for the additional lifting power that reduces deposition of color.

Formulation of a liquid tint with 20 volume cream peroxide often does not create a solution strong enough to achieve good coverage. The additives and thickeners in cream peroxide can buffer the strength of the liquid tint formula to the extent that complete coverage does not occur on resistant gray hair.

HYDROGEN PEROXIDE VOLUME COMPARISON

EXPERIMENT INSTRUCTION SHEET

Objectives

To observe and document the results when processing non-pigmented hair with permanent tints formulated with varying volumes of peroxide. To gain experience formulating with a variety of volumes.

Hair Swatches Needed

4 non-pigmented hair swatches (either 100 percent or salt and pepper) from the same head cutting

Labeling Hair Swatches

Label the hair swatches to indicate the level of hydrogen peroxide that will be used on each.

- 10 volume H_2O_2
- 20 volume H_2O_2
- 30 volume H_2O_2
- 40 volume H_2O_2

Materials Needed

- Level 5 or 6 tint
- Hydrogen peroxide—10, 20, 30, and 40 volume
- Nonmetallic mixing receptacles

Procedure

1. Mix ½ teaspoon of each tint with each individual volume of hydrogen peroxide in nonmetallic mixing receptacles.
2. Thoroughly saturate swatches with various tint strengths as indicated on labels.
3. Process each strand for 55 minutes. (Remember that standard processing time on non-pigmented hair is 45 minutes. The extra 10 minutes simulates the application time on an entire head.)
4. Shampoo, rinse, and dry each swatch.
5. Mount swatches on the *Experiment Results Sheet on page R-129.*
6. Answer the *Review Questions on page R-131.*

PRESOFTENING EXTREMELY RESISTANT HAIR

Occasionally gray hair is so resistant that even when formulation, application, and timing are correct, coverage is not satisfactory and presoftening becomes necessary. Presoftening is a two-step or double application hair coloring in which two distinct and separate applications of product are necessary to achieve the desired shade. The presoftener is applied, processed, and removed. The second step is the application of the tint to complete the two-step coloring process.

The purpose of presoftening is twofold: to soften and open the cuticle for improved penetration of color and to create missing yellow or gold tones in the hair so that the tint with a balance of color will adhere and process on-tone.

In the past, presoftening was done prior to most oxidation hair coloring services to open the cuticle and allow penetration to the cortex. Technology has created colors that have presoftening agents in the formulation, making presoftening necessary only in cases of very resistant gray hair.

The order of resistance determines whether or not hair will need presoftening prior to tinting.

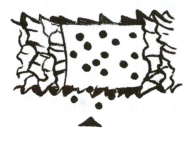

Permanent color quickly and easily penetrates the raised cuticle layers of bleached hair.

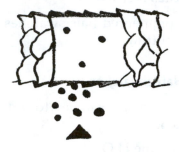

The tight cuticle layers of naturally gray hair resist penetration.

LIQUID PRESOFTENERS

Formulation of a Liquid Presoftener

The most common form of presoftener used in the past, and still used today for its economy, is a mixture of one ounce of 20 volume hydrogen peroxide and eight drops of 28 percent ammonia water.

Liquid Presoftener Application Procedure

1. Dip cotton applicator into presoftener and squeeze out excess so as not to drip in client's eyes or face.
2. Dab, do not rub, the liquid presoftener onto the resistant areas.
3. Process at room temperature for 5-10 minutes.
4. Towel blot.
5. Apply tint.

CREAM PRESOFTENERS

Gold based tints, oil and cream bleaches can be used as cream presofteners. All will work to soften and open the cuticle. However, a gold base tint will deposit yellow or gold into the hair while a bleach will only diffuse and oxidize the remaining natural pigment within the shaft.

Formulation of Cream Presofteners

Follow the standard manufacturer's recommended directions to mix either an oil bleach or a lifting tint. However, if using a cream bleach, use no protinator, activator, or catalyst. White or gray hair does not require high lift and to do so will only cause unnecessary damage.

Cream Presoftener Application Procedure

1. Mix product according to manufacturer's directions.
2. Apply with brush or bottle in most resistant areas first.
3. Process at room temperature for 5-20 minutes.
4. Rinse thoroughly and shampoo.
5. Apply tint.

PRESOFTENING COMPARISON

EXPERIMENT INSTRUCTION SHEET

Objectives

To gain experience in mixing the various formulations available for presoftening of resistant hair. To compare the results achieved with these different products.

Hair Swatches Needed

- 4 *thick* white or gray hair swatches
- 4 *thick* salt-and-pepper hair swatches

Labeling Hair Swatches

Label one white or gray swatch and one salt-and-pepper swatch each as follows:
- Liquid presoftener
- Oil bleach
- Cream bleach
- Tint

Materials Needed

- 20 volume hydrogen peroxide
- Oil bleach
- Cream bleach
- 28% ammonia water
- Gold based tint

Formulation

1. *Liquid presoftener:*
   - ¼ ounce 20 volume hydrogen peroxide
   - 2 drops of 28 percent ammonia water
2. *Cream presofteners:*
   - Oil bleach: 1 teaspoon bleach, two teaspoons H_2O_2.
   - Cream bleach: 1 teaspoon bleach, two teaspoons H_2O_2.
   - Gold tint: 1 teaspoon tint plus appropriate amount of H_2O_2.

Application

1. Thoroughly saturate each swatch as indicated on its label.
2. Process at room temperature for 15 minutes. (5-10 minutes is normal processing time. The extra 5 minutes simulates application time.)
3. Shampoo, rinse, and dry each swatch at the end of 15 minutes.
4. Cut half of the hair out of each swatch. Glue and tape the end for use in the next experiment.
5. Label each new swatch as to the natural color and which presoftener was applied and use for experiment *Tinting Presoftened Hair.*.
6. Mount swatches on the *Experiment Results Sheet on page R-133.*
6. Answer the *Review Questions on page R-135.*

TINTING PRESOFTENED HAIR
EXPERIMENT INSTRUCTION SHEET

Objectives

To observe and document the color results achieved when tinting over gray, white, and salt-and-pepper hair that has been presoftened with four different presofteners.

Hair Swatches Needed

This experiment is performed on the half of each swatch that was treated with presoftener and then removed from the previous experiment comparing the four presoftening products.

Labeling Hair Swatches

Swatches should already be labeled from the presoftening experiment as to their natural color and product used.

Materials Needed

- 20 volume hydrogen peroxide
- Level 5—Neutral medium brown tint

Procedure

1. Mix ¼ ounce of tint with the appropriate amount of 20 volume hydrogen peroxide.
2. Thoroughly saturate each swatch.
3. Process at room temperature for 55 minutes. (Remember that standard processing time on non-pigmented hair is 45 minutes. The extra 10 minutes simulates the application time on an entire head.)
4. Shampoo, rinse, and dry each swatch.
5. Mount swatches on the *Experiment Results Sheet on page R-137.*
6. Answer the *Review Questions on page R-139.*

AVOIDING PRESOFTENING

On a truly resistant head of gray hair, presoftening sometimes can be avoided by scheduling the retouch applications every three weeks instead of monthly. At three week intervals the keratin will not have hardened as much as it will in four weeks, and therefore, the color can penetrate easier. The following check list details other techniques for achieving satisfactory gray coverage before resorting to a two-step process (presoftening and tinting):

1. Waxes in makeup can inhibit the penetration of hair color. In this case, shampoo and thoroughly dry the hair before application.
2. Apply product rapidly so that it is strong enough to process as intended by the manufacturer.
3. Process a full 45 minutes for complete coverage.
4. Use a generous amount of product, particularly around the hairline. These fine hairs tend to dry out before processing is complete.
5. Apply color against the cuticle growth to push color under the cuticle for improved penetration.
6. Lift and separate hair away from the scalp to allow air to circulate.
7. Add more warmth to the formula.
8. Add more depth to the formula.

100 PERCENT COVERAGE

You've probably heard the old saying, "Be careful what you ask for, because you just might get it." Beware of asking for 100 percent coverage. When every hair is exactly the same color, the result is often flat and lacking life, like a painted wall. The blending of colors that is achieved when every hair is not colored is softer and more flattering than 100 percent coverage.

COLOR WASHING

When only a hint of color is desired, color washing can tone without a drastic change or definite line of regrowth. Color washing can be done on white or solid gray hair to give just a hint of color change or it can be done on salt-and-pepper hair with a color that is close to the shade of the remaining pigmented hair. The formula for this service would be:

- 1 ounce tint
- 1 ounce 10 volume hydrogen peroxide

Apply this mixture with the soap cap method to clean damp hair. The timing would be approximately 15-20 minutes at room temperature for normal hair or 10 minutes for delicate or chemically treated hair.

COLORING A NON-PIGMENTED STREAK

To tone a gray or white streak with a temporary color of a light shade causes no special problems. Temporary colors contain no oxidizer to affect the dark hair. However, the dark shades are not designed to cover gray or white hair. The dark shades are designed to be applied to hair that already has a strong color base, and thus tend to grab the base color of the rinse when used on non-pigmented hair.

Most semipermanent colors are efficient for enhancing, toning, or covering gray streaks. They are easy to apply because even if the semipermanent color touches the natural hair, no harm is done.

More care and special consideration must be given when using a penetrating tint. When toning the gray or white streak to a color that is lighter than the natural color, care must be taken *not* to allow the tint to touch the darker hair. A toning or lightening tint will bring out the brass in the virgin hair. When tinting the gray or white streak to a color that will match the dark hair, the tint must be left on the strand for 45 minutes for complete coverage. To blend the color and break any line of demarcation, work color through surrounding hair for only a few minutes. Remember, color on color makes a darker color. Therefore, if the tint remains on the dark hair for 45 minutes, the overall look will be much darker than the natural shade of hair.

If the streak is resistant, use any of the methods described for use on an entire head of resistant hair. However, be sure to control the product as a presoftener that touches the natural hair may cause brass and spots.

10

Kinetic Molecular Theory of Lightening

One of the most frequent questions a colorist asks when lightening is "Where does the color go?" It cannot be seen washing down the drain when the bleach is removed, nor does it appear to be absorbed into the bleach. In the early 60's many cosmetologists were told that the bleaching agent "ate" the natural pigment. This theory was demonstrated and "proved" by the addition of a bottle of tint to a bleach formula. The colored tint would disappear before your very eyes!

The advancement of science and the development of high-powered microscopes that could actually "see" down into the hair shaft have proven that our first theories were incorrect. Technology has brought the Kinetic Molecular Theory of Lightening.

The Kinetic (pronounced kin-ET-ic) Molecular Theory explains that gases consist of tiny, discrete molecules. These molecules are relatively far apart with empty space between them. All the molecules within a gas are constantly in rapid motion, moving in straight lines until they collide with other molecules.

This constant movement causes the molecules to sometimes crash into each other with enough force to break apart atoms. When atoms are set free by such a collision, they can join with other free atoms to form new compounds.

The gases that are released by the addition of hydrogen peroxide to a bleach formula, a process known as oxidation, create this kinetic motion within the cortical layer of the hair shaft. The gases crash into the melanin or pigment with enough force to diffuse (break apart and spread out) the molecules of color. The free oxygen atom that oxidizes the melanin within the hair shaft is the result of this collision between molecules in the lightening product and the natural pigment of the hair.

Heat increases the kinetic action within any compound. The oxidation process that is occurring within the bleach formula causes heat and this chemical heat is enhanced by the body heat. Therefore, the stronger the chemical formula and the closer it is placed to the scalp, the greater the diffusion of melanin within the shaft.

Decreasing the volume of the gas shortens the average distance between the molecules and thereby increases the number of collisions per unit time. As soon as hydrogen peroxide is mixed into the bleach formula, it begins to release oxygen and the volume decreases. This process continues until the product either dries out or releases all available oxygen molecules.

Manufacturers of lighteners implement the Kinetic Molecular Theory in different degrees or strengths in a variety of formulas, but all diffuse, rather than remove, color, as previously believed. The eye interprets this diffusion of color, whether within the hair shaft or in a bowl of bleach to which tint has been added, as a lighter shade. This diffusion of color will occur before your very eyes in the next color experiment!

KINETIC MOLECULAR THEORY

EXPERIMENT INSTRUCTION SHEET

Objectives

To observe and document the Kinetic Molecular Theory as it applies to color diffusion.

Materials Needed

- Powder bleach
- Black tint
- Gloves
- Measuring device
- Nonmetallic mixing receptacle
- 20 volume liquid or cream hydrogen peroxide

Procedure

1. Place 1 tablespoon of powder bleach in the mixing receptacle.
2. Stir in enough liquid or cream 20 volume hydrogen peroxide to make a creamy paste.
3. To this mixture, add ¼ teaspoon of black tint.
4. Answer the *Review Questions on page R-141.*

HISTORY OF HAIR LIGHTENING

The illustrious history of hair lightening began in ancient Rome. A natural blonde was a rare sight in this predominantly dark-haired nation. To avoid confusion and misunderstandings on the streets of Rome, the state decreed that "ladies of the evening" would be required by law to lighten their hair to blonde or wear a yellow wig.

Valeria Messalina, third wife of Emperor Claudius, caused quite a stir and led what might have been the first organized women's liberation movement. Valeria took great pleasure in donning a yellow wig and tiptoeing out into the night to masquerade as one of the girls for hire. However, few were fooled, as she often returned to the palace without her wig. Valeria Messalina was the talk of the town, but she did leave her mark on fashion history as respectable women rushed to have their hair bleached or to purchase yellow wigs. Valeria may have been the inspiration behind the slogan "Blondes have more fun."

Colorists of the early 1900's used a mixture of hydrogen peroxide and a few drops of ammonia to lighten the hair. White henna (powdered magnesium carbonate) or soap flakes were added to thicken the mixture. This formula did not offer a great variety of lightening possibilities to the colorist or client.

THE THREE CLASSIFICATIONS OF BLEACH:
OIL, CREAM, AND POWDER

Today's colorists have at their disposal three basic classifications of bleach. Each classification has unique uses, abilities, chemical characteristics, and formulation procedures.

Oil Bleach

Oil bleaches are the mildest of the three types and have the least amount of lightening action. This product is appropriate when only one or two levels of color lift are desired. Oil bleach can be used as a single-application color to achieve a moderate color change of the entire head or in weaving or streaking to achieve a very subtle color change. It is also a popular product for presoftening resistant gray hair prior to a tinting service. Because oil bleach is so mild, it is used professionally to lighten excessively dark facial and body hair.

Chemical Composition of Oil Bleach

Oil bleach is a shampoo based product. The shampoo serves to facilitate easy removal when the lightening service is complete. Sulfonated oils (oils treated with sulfuric acid or castor oil) are added to the bleach to slow down the bleaching action. This is the same type of oil that is used to make soapless shampoo.

Oil bleaches contain a weak hydrogen peroxide and ammonia solution. This solution creates an alkaline pH strong enough to soften and open the cuticle layer of the hair shaft allowing the bleach to gently lighten the hair color.

Cream Bleach

The cream bleaches are strong enough to do pastel blonding, yet gentle enough to be used on the scalp. Cream bleach will take hair through the "Seven Stages of Lightening," which are: black, brown, red, red-gold, gold, yellow, and pale yellow.

Chemical Composition of Cream Bleach

Cream bleaches are similar to oil bleaches in that both have a shampoo base containing sulfonated oil. Nonyl nonoxynol-10 is a nonionic surfactant used to make the shampoo base of many cream bleaches. Ethyl hydroxymethyl oleyl oxazoline and PEG-5, short for polyethylene glycol/polyoxyethylene, are waxes also used to make the nonionic surfactants that comprise this shampoo base. They serve to make the product resistant to hard water, dissolve in oil, and spread easily. These nonionic surfactants have no known toxicity.

Tall oil acid and oleic acid are both oils used in cream bleaches and also double as pH adjusters. Tall oil acid is a dark brown liquid by-product of the pinewood pulp industry. It also works as a fungicide. Tall oil can be a mild irritant and sensitizer. Oleic acid is taken from animal and vegetable fats and oils and has better penetrating abilities than many other oils. Like tall oil, oleic acid can be a mild irritant.

Soyamine is another oil used in cream bleach. A derivative of soybean oil, soyamine is also used in the manufacture of soaps, shampoos, bath oils, margarine, and other foods. Soybean oil has been known to cause allergic reactions that include pimples and hair damage.

Cream bleaches generally contain 3 percent ammonia. Ammonium hydroxide is the technical name for ammonia water, but it is commonly known as hartshorn, spirits of hartshorn, or aqua ammonia. The chemical symbol for ammonia is NH_3. This weak alkali is a colorless, pungent gas composed of hydrogen and nitrogen. The 3 percent ammonia creates within the product an alkaline pH strong enough to soften and open the cuticle layer of the hair shaft. A formula that contains more than 3 percent can speed up the bleaching action to the point that the damage to the hair cannot be controlled.

Cream bleaches have an average pH of 10 and contain a solution of hydrogen peroxide that may be as great as 3 percent. This is strong enough to enhance the softening abilities of the bleach without oxidizing it within the shipping container.

Hydrochloric acid is a clear liquid used to speed up the oxidation process. This ingredient is partly responsible for the warning not to sniff bleach products as the fumes can cause inflammation of the respiratory tract.

Isopropyl alcohol is added as an antibacterial, a solvent, and to give the product such a bad taste that no one will consider ingesting it. Prepared from petroleum, isopropyl alcohol is also found in hair-color rinses, hand lotions, many cosmetics, antifreeze, and shellac.

Ethoxydiglycol is a liquid solvent similar to isopropyl alcohol. This derivative of petroleum is also used as a solvent and thinner in nail enamels. It is toxic to animals but no specific human data is now available. It is non-irritating and non-penetrating on human skin.

Ethylene glycol is also used as a solvent and humectant in cream bleaches as well as antifreeze.

In addition, many cream bleaches contain conditioners. Studies indicate that bleaches containing protein give the hair slightly better manageability, less brittleness, and more fiber strength than lighteners lacking the additive.

To further protect the hair, emollients and humectants such as lauryl alcohol and oleyl alcohol are often added. Lauryl alcohol is a colorless crystal produced from coconut oil. It has good sudsing ability and is soluble in the oils used in cream bleaches. Oleyl alcohol, under the registered trade name of Ocenol, is an oily yellow compound found in fish oil.

Also found in most cream bleaches is a clouding agent and a thickener for easier control. The clouding agent makes the cream bleach easier to see on the hair shaft than the oil bleach while the thickener increases the product's ability to stay where it was placed on the shaft.

Many manufacturers add a drabber to reduce brassy tones. Green, blue, and violet are effective because these are the tones on the Chromatic Circle that neutralize the red, orange, and yellow tones which naturally occur as the melanin goes through the Seven Stages of Lightening. Other manufacturers prefer to leave their bleach a pure white in color so that the colorist can monitor the lightening process without wiping the product off.

Trideth-6 or tridecyl alcohol is a paraffin obtained from petroleum that is used in cream bleach to keep the product blended and prevent separation.

Ethylenediamine tetraacetic acid (EDTA) is added for its ability to preserve the color, texture, and appearance of cream bleaches. It is found in many beauty products, especially shampoo. While EDTA has been used in the past in carbonated beverages, it is suspected to cause cancer.

Fragrance is one of the last items on the ingredient list, meaning that only a small portion of the formula is devoted to making the product more pleasant to smell. Most colorists would testify that the percentage of fragrance is too small to be of much benefit.

Protinators/Activators

Protinators are used to increase lifting power. Protinator, activator, booster, and catalyst are all terms used to designate the dry crystal that is added to cream bleach to create a stronger product. The greater the number of protinators, the greater the strength of the formula.

- 0 activator—formula comparable to oil bleach in mildness
- 1 activator—will lighten light brown hair
- 2 activators—will lighten medium to dark brown hair
- 3 activators—will lighten resistant dark brown hair
- 4 activators—equivalent of powder bleach. Not used on scalp.

Chemical Composition of Protinators/Activators

Silica is a thickening agent used so that when the hydrogen peroxide and cream bleach are added, a paste is formed that is easier to apply and evaporates slower, allowing the lightener to work for longer periods of time. Silica is not harmful to the skin and hair while wet, but draws moisture out as it dries.

Sodium lauryl sulfate is often added to make the product easier to spread, to remove oils from the shaft, and as a wetting agent. Sodium lauryl sulfate, like silica, is generally nontoxic, but can dry the skin and hair.

An alkali, such as sodium metasilicate, is added to neutralize the acid in the hydrogen peroxide. Sodium metasilicate is made from sand and soda ash. It is also used in the manufacture of detergents.

Boosters are included to destabilize or activate the hydrogen peroxide. The manufacturer's recommended amount of booster has the effect of doubling the strength of the hydrogen peroxide solution.

Urea peroxide, potassium persulfate, and ammonium persulfate are examples of compounds that make up the booster characteristics of activators. Urea hydrogen peroxide is a white crystal or powder derived from urea. Ammonium persulfate is a colorless crystal that increases the oxidation and leaves the hair dry and brittle if overused. Potassium sulfate is a colorless crystal that doubles as a salt substitute.

Colored toners, such as D & C violet no. 2, are added to protinators in an effort to drab out unwanted brassiness as the melanin is diffused within the hair shaft.

Disodium EDTA is a preservative that prevents color and texture changes in the product. EDTA is a controversial ingredient because it is suspected of causing cancer in laboratory animals.

Powder Bleaches

Powder bleaches, like cream bleaches, are strong enough to do pastel blonding. However, powder bleach *cannot* be applied to the scalp because it does not contain the oil and conditioners that make a cream bleach safe for on-the-scalp application. Application to the scalp would result in severe skin irritation and possibly chemical burns. Powder bleach is used exclusively for off-the-scalp applications, such as frosting, foil-wrapped weaving, highlighting with plastic cups, and hair painting.

Chemical Composition of Powder Bleaches

Like oil and cream bleaches, powder bleaches contain ammonia. In this instance, however, it is in a dry form. The ammonia begins the oxidation process when it mixes with liquid or cream hydrogen peroxide.

The chemical formula for powder bleach usually includes a type of "activator" that speeds up the release of oxygen from hydrogen peroxide. Ammonium percarbonate, sodium peroxide, and ammonium persulfate are examples of compounds added to powder bleach for this purpose.

Ammonium persulfate (ammonium salt) works as an oxidizer in dyes as well as bleaches and also has disinfecting, deodorizing, and preserving abilities. Ammonium persulfate is irritating to the skin and mucous membranes and can leave the hair brittle.

Potassium sulfate is a colorless or white crystal that also acts as an oxidizer in powder bleach formulas and doubles as a solvent to dissolve water-insoluble compounds on and in the hair shaft. Potassium sulfate is also an ingredient in salt substitutes and fertilizer.

Urea peroxide is an odorless, crystal product created from protein metabolism that is present in the urine of all carnivorous animals. Urea serves many purposes in the beauty industry, such as in shampoos, roll-on deodorants, mouthwashes, and semipermanent colors, but the use to consider at this time is its ability to boost the power of hydrogen peroxide.

The amount of urea peroxide contained in a bleach differs from manufacturer to manufacturer. However, because it is an ingredient that has a volume of its own, it is crucial to consider when mixing the formula. The potential for danger occurs when a solution of hydrogen peroxide with more than 20 volume is added to the bleach. Because urea peroxide has a volume of its own, the addition of 20 volume peroxide increases, rather than decreases, the working volume of the product as it goes on the scalp and hair.

Sodium metasilicate is an alkali made from soda ash and sand that creates the alkaline pH base of powder bleach. It is also used in detergents and to preserve eggs in egg shampoo. Sodium metasilicate is caustic, meaning that it can burn skin.

Sodium chloride, found on the ingredients list of some powder bleaches, is common table salt. It is a white odorless crystal that has the ability to absorb moisture. While the bleach solution is moist, it does not irritate the skin, but upon drying it pulls water from the skin and this can cause irritation.

Ethyl cellulose works to bind the ingredients of the bleach together and make it easy to spread on the hair shaft. Ethyl cellulose, while not a form of colorant itself, is used in many coloring products and cosmetics to facilitate the work of the colorants.

Hydroxypropyl methylcellulose is used in the formula to give a thick, sticky consistency when the bleach is mixed with liquid peroxide. It is resistant to bacteria and has no known toxicity.

Aluminum stearate or aluminum tristearate is a hard plastic material that is also used to thicken powder bleaches. It is commonly used in colorants, cosmetics, chewing gum, and as a waterproofing for fabrics.

Silica is a coloring agent that occurs naturally in many rocks. Sand is silica. Silicones are made from silica and used in many beauty products such as protective cream, hair-waving preparations, straighteners, and hand lotions. Sometimes this ingredient is listed as hydrated silica, which means the silica has been combined with water.

Tetrasodium EDTA, disodium EDTA, and sodium edetate are powdered sodium salts that work as sequestering agents and chelating agents in many powder bleaches. As a sequestering agent, tetrasodium EDTA works as a preservative to prevent physical and chemical changes affecting the color, texture, and appearance of the product. Both the sequestering and chelating properties of this ingredient help to prevent adverse reaction when the bleach comes in contact with metal or metallic salts.

Sorbitol is a texturizer and humectant used to preserve the moisture content of the mixture. It is widely used as a replacement for glycerin in mouthwashes, dental creams, embalming fluid, antifreeze, and a variety of cosmetics and hair coloring agents. It is found in many berries, and because of its sweet taste is used in foods as a sugar substitute.

Magnesium carbonate is a fragrance carrier and coloring agent that is used in many beauty products other than powder bleach. It is commonly found on the ingredient list of baby, bath, face, and tooth powder, face masks and dry rouge. Non-beauty items that use magnesium carbonate are paint, table salt, printing ink, and antacids. It is available in both natural and artificial form. Magnesium carbonate is nontoxic to the unbroken skin but may be quite irritating if applied over an abrasion.

Sodium lauryl sulfate is a surfactant included in bleach to assist with the removal of the product. It also works as a wetting agent and to hold the ingredients of the mixture together. Sodium lauryl sulfate can be drying to the skin because it is a degreaser.

A great variety of pigments, such as ultramarine blue, FD&C blue no. 1 aluminum lake, are added to powdered bleach to "drab" the brassy tones that appear as the hair goes through the seven stages of lightening.

THREE CLASSIFICATIONS OF BLEACHES

EXPERIMENT INSTRUCTION SHEET

Objectives

To observe and document the various strengths of bleaches used on virgin hair, and the differences in the degree of lightening achieved.

Hair Swatches Needed

3 virgin hair swatches (brown or black) from the same head cutting.

Labeling Hair Swatches

Label individual swatches:
- Oil bleach
- Cream bleach
- Powder bleach

Materials Needed

- Cream bleach
- Oil bleach
- Powder bleach
- 20 volume liquid H_2O_2
- 20 volume cream H_2O_2
- Activators/protinators

Formulation

1. *Oil Bleach Formula:*
   - ½ teaspoon oil bleach
   - 1 teaspoon liquid 20 volume H_2O_2
2. *Cream Bleach Formula:*
   - ½ ounce liquid 20 volume hydrogen peroxide
   - ⅛ of the manufacturer's recommended measurement of activator/protinator
   - ¼ ounce cream bleach
3. *Powder Bleach:*
   - 1 teaspoon powder bleach
   - Cream or liquid 20 volume hydrogen peroxide to make a creamy paste

Procedure

1. Saturate the 3 swatches with the bleach indicated on label.
2. Process 45 minutes at room temperature.
3. Shampoo, rinse, and dry swatches thoroughly.
4. Mount swatches on the *Experiment Results Sheet on page R-143.*
5. Answer the *Review Questions on page R-145.*

PHYSICAL AND CHEMICAL CHANGES OF LIGHTENING

Even the darkest black hair can be lightened to pale yellow. *(See Color Plate 29.)* However, there will be many chemical and physical changes in the hair during the process. The first physical change that the hair will go through is a succession of colors known as the:

SEVEN STAGES OF LIGHTENING

Stage 1—Black
Stage 2—Brown
Stage 3—Red
Stage 4—Red-gold
Stage 5—Gold
Stage 6—Yellow
Stage 7—Pale yellow

Another structural change is that the texture of the hair becomes coarser. Lighteners cause the shaft to swell and lift the cuticle layer to allow penetration to the cortex. When the lightener is removed and the pH of the shaft is restored to normal, the shaft shrinks back down toward its prior size, but never quite reaches it. Some of the cuticle layer remains raised and thus each strand of hair becomes "fatter" or coarser.

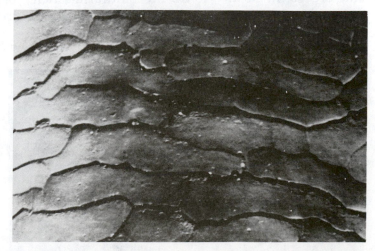

Cuticle layers of healthy virgin hair are smooth and fit together tightly, like scales on a fish. (Courtesy: Redken Laboratories, Inc.)

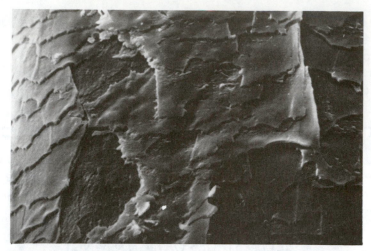

Bleaching causes the cuticle layers to swell, becoming raised and roughened.
(Courtesy: Redken Laboratories, Inc.)

Another structural change occurs with the breaking and restructuring of cortical bonds within the shaft. The weakening of these bonds makes the hair more pliable and less resistant. This additional pliability is considered an asset especially in conjunction with competition hair styling, fingerwaving, sculpture curling, roller setting, and backcombing.

The elasticity of the hair is also altered by lightening, and especially by bleaching. It is the most crucial factor to monitor during the lightening process. Healthy hair will stretch approximately 1/5 of its length and then bounce back to normal. Lightening makes changes in this ability that are apparent, yet appear different depending on whether the hair is wet or dry.

If the hair is over-lightened, moist strands will stretch more than 1/5 of their hair length and not bounce back. They can even be stretched to the point where the hair snaps and breaks. In its dry form, the natural elasticity of over-lightened hair will appear to be decreased. In fact, in this condition, the hair becomes dry, brittle, and can snap just from normal combing and brushing.

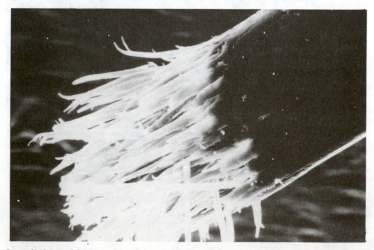

Over-lightened hair ends split and fray.   (Courtesy: Redken Laboratories, Inc.)

With each level of color lift, the hair will exhibit signs of increased dryness, porosity, and pliability. The dryness is easily treated with moisturizers, and the porosity is treated with protein treatments so that the hair retains the benefits of increased pliability without becoming excessively dry, elastic, or porous.

Most heads of healthy hair can be safely lifted to the pale blonde stage. It is the job of the professional colorist to analyze the hair prior to lightening, and to closely observe the stages of lightening to determine how light the color can be taken. Performing a preliminary test strand takes the guess work out of this procedure.

The hair is never safely lifted past the pale yellow stage to a white with bleach. The extreme diffusion of color necessary to give a white appearance to the eye causes excessive damage to the cuticle and cortex, and sometimes even the medulla. The result is that wet hair feels "mushy" and will stretch without returning to its original length. When dry, the hair will be harsh and brittle. Such hair often suffers breakage and will not accept a toner properly. However, this does *not* mean that only those born with blonde hair can be a white blonde. The baby-blonde look can be achieved by lightening to pale yellow and neutralizing with a toner. This process is explained further in the sections titled *Creating a Foundation for Toners on page 152* and *Toners on page 153.*

SEVEN STAGES OF LIGHTENING

EXPERIMENT INSTRUCTION SHEET

Objectives

To observe and document the Seven Stages of Lightening that occur as hair of the darkest stage is taken to the lightest stage of color within the realm of safe bleaching.

Hair Swatches Needed

7 black hair swatches that have not received prior permanent coloring treatments

Labeling Hair Swatches

Label the hair swatches to indicate the stage of color to be achieved on each individual strand:

- Stage 1—Black
- Stage 2—Brown
- Stage 3—Red
- Stage 4—Red-gold
- Stage 5—Gold
- Stage 6—Yellow
- Stage 7—Pale yellow

Materials Needed

- Powder bleach
- Oil bleach
- 20 volume H_2O_2

Procedure

1. Do *not* apply bleach to the swatch labeled "black." It is to remain virgin to illustrate the darkest stage of color.
2. Apply oil bleach to stage 2—brown swatch. (Powder bleach will lighten past the brown stage too quickly to control it.)
3. Thoroughly saturate the remaining swatches with powder bleach.
4. Begin timing. The darkest levels will be achieved first. Each swatch will reach the desired shade of lift and be ready for product removal at a different time.
5. Shampoo, rinse, and dry each swatch as they reach the desired level of lightness.
6. Mount swatches on the *Experiment Results Sheet on page R-147.*
7. Answer the *Review Questions on page R-149.*

ACTIVATOR COMPARISON

EXPERIMENT INSTRUCTION SHEET

Objectives

To observe and document the difference in the lightening abilities of cream bleach when it is mixed without activators/protinators or with either one, two, three, or four activators. To observe and document which formulation offers the appropriate strength and speed to decolorize light, medium, or dark virgin hair.

Hair Swatches Needed

5 virgin brown hair swatches from the same head cutting.

Labeling Hair Swatches

Label swatches as follows:

- 0 activator
- 1 activator
- 2 activators
- 3 activators
- 4 activators

Materials Needed

- Cream bleach with activators or protinators
- 20 volume liquid hydrogen peroxide

Formulation

1. *0 Activator Formula*
   - ½ ounce cream bleach
   - 1 ounce liquid 20 volume H_2O_2

2. *1 Activator Formula*
   - 1 ounce liquid 20 volume H_2O_2
   - ¼ package activator
   - ½ ounce cream bleach

3. *2 Activator Formula*
   - 1 ounce liquid 20 volume H_2O_2
   - ½ package activator
   - ½ ounce cream bleach

4. *3 Activator Formula*
   - 1 ounce liquid 20 volume H_2O_2
   - ¾ package activator
   - ½ ounce cream bleach

5. *4 Activator Formula*
   - 1 ounce liquid 20 volume H_2O_2
   - 1 package activator
   - ½ ounce cream bleach

Procedure

1. Process swatches each for 1 hour at room temperature.
2. Shampoo, rinse, and dry swatches thoroughly
3. Mount swatches on the *Experiment Results Sheet on page R-151.*
4. Answer the *Review Questions on page R-153.*

TIME FACTORS: LEVEL, TONE, PRODUCT STRENGTH, AND ARTIFICIAL HEAT

The darker the natural color of the hair, the more melanin it has. The more melanin it has, the longer it takes to diffuse the color to give a lighter appearance to the hair. The amount of time needed to lighten the natural color is also influenced by the porosity. Porous hair of the same color level will lighten faster than hair that is nonporous because the bleaching agent can enter the cortex more rapidly.

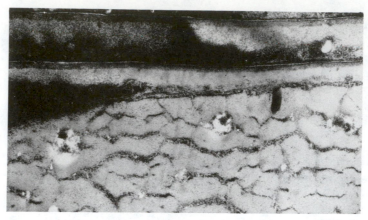

This virgin brown hair was saturated with a medium strength bleach for 1 hour. The diffusion of pigment has left air pockets where the melanin molecules once were.   (Courtesy: Redken Laboratories, Inc.)

Tone also influences the length of time necessary to lighten the natural hair color. The greater the percentage of red reflected in the natural color, the more difficult it is to achieve the pale, delicate shades of blonde. The ash blondes are especially difficult to achieve because the melanin must be diffused sufficiently to alter both the level and tone of the hair.

The strength of the product also effects the speed and amount of lightening. The stronger bleaches achieve the pale shades in the least amount of time.

The application of heat to any bleach will speed up its lightening abilities by increasing the natural motion of the molecules as explained by the Kinetic Molecular Theory. The higher the temperature, the greater the motion of the molecules. Because heat, used in conjunction with lightening chemicals, softens the hair, creating a fragile state, caution must be exercised when using heat. Excessive heat can cause the motion of the molecules to become so great that extreme damage can occur as cuticle layers are removed and cortical bonds are destroyed.

By increasing kinetic activity, heat leads to quicker lightening, thus shortening the time needed for decolorization. The stages of lightening must be carefully observed to avoid excessive lift that could lead to the diffusion of so much natural pigment that the desired toner shade may not develop properly in the hair shaft. When this occurs, the toner may "grab" the base color, giving the hair an ashy, gray tone. However, beautiful blondes can safely be achieved on anyone with proper analysis, products, and techniques.

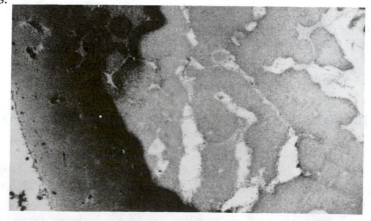

This strand has been overbleached. This excessive diffusion of natural pigment will not create the proper foundation for toner development.   (Courtesy: Redken Laboratories, Inc.)

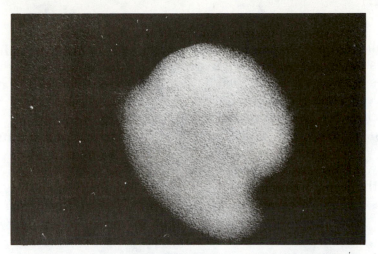

This air pocket was once filled with one large molecule of melanin. After 2 hours of bleaching, the pigment is diffused to the outer edges of the air pocket.   (Courtesy: Redken Laboratories, Inc.)

EFFECTS OF ARTIFICIAL HEAT ON BLEACH

EXPERIMENT INSTRUCTION SHEET

Objectives

To observe and document the effects of heat on the three classifications of bleaches.

Hair Swatches Needed

6 brown hair swatches that have not received prior permanent coloring treatments.

Labeling Hair Swatches

Label as follows:

- Oil bleach—artificial heat
- Oil bleach—no heat
- Cream bleach—artificial heat
- Cream bleach—no heat
- Powder bleach—artificial heat
- Powder bleach—no heat

Materials Needed

- Oil bleach
- Powder bleach
- Cream bleach with activators or protinators
- 20 volume liquid hydrogen peroxide
- Plastic or potato wrap

Procedure

1. Mix small amounts of each bleach according to manufacturer's directions.
2. Swatches labeled "no heat" are to process naturally.
3. Swatches labeled "artificial heat" are to be wrapped in plastic or potato wrap and processed under a warm dryer.
4. All swatches are to be processed for 20 minutes.
5. Shampoo, rinse, and dry each swatch at the end of the 20 minute processing time.
6. Mount swatches on the *Experiment Results Sheet on page R-155*.
7. Answer the *Review Questions on page R-157*.

CREATING A FOUNDATION FOR TONING

The secret to successful toning to white and every other shade of blonde is to create the correct "foundation" during the pre-lightening process. As hair color goes through the Seven Stages of Lightening, the color remaining in the shaft is known as the "foundation." The colorist may remove the lightener and chose to leave behind a foundation of gold, pale yellow, or any of the other stages.

Most manufacturers publish literature identifying the foundation recommended to achieve the intended results with a particular toner. The foundation stage achieved through pre-lightening is crucial to proper processing of the second step of a two-step color.

If the hair is over-lightened, removing the correct foundation, the tint or toner used will tend to "grab" the base color, processing both darker and cooler than the expected shade. If the hair is not pre-lightened enough, the amount of pigment in the tint or toner will be insufficient to correct the brassiness that occurred as a result of the diffusion of the melanin.

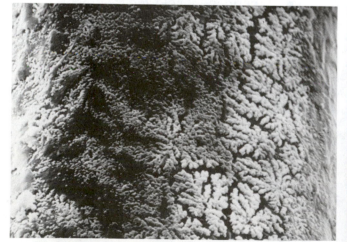 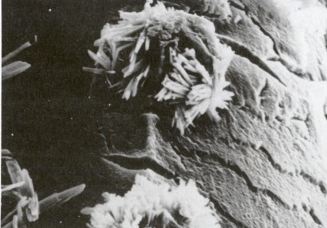

Both of these strands of hair have been prebleached and then coated to correct overporosity in preparation for toning. (Courtesy: Redken Laboratories, Inc.)

TONERS

Saturation of color is the prime difference between a toner and a tint. A toner is a permanent aniline derivative hair coloring just as is a tint. However, the dye load is a smaller percentage of the formula which creates pale delicate shades of color that are used to "tone" pre-lightened hair. Use of a pre-lightener and toner is the classic example of a double-process color (also known as a two-step tint or a double-application color).

Pre-lightening creates the foundation for correct development of the pastel blonde toners. The paler the toner, the lighter the foundation stage must be. Without pre-lightening, a toner will not develop to the shade indicated on the color chart.

In addition to the correct stage, the colorist must consider the porosity of the hair shaft. Because of these variables, it is important for the colorist to experiment with toner development on swatches before performing the service on clients.

Pre-lightening creates the additional porosity necessary for color development. Occasionally a naturally blonde head of hair may reach the correct color foundation without achieving sufficient porosity.

Even hair that is naturally lighter than the shade of the toner and appears light enough to accept the color will not develop correctly until the porosity is created to allow penetration of the toner. Therefore, even when toning gray or white hair, the hair must be pre-lightened.

Chemical Composition

Other than the reduced dye load, the chemical ingredients and chemical action of a toner are the same as a tint.

Color Selection

Toners are available in warm, cool, and neutral shades just as are the tints. The Artist's Concept of the Laws of Color is the basis for formulating and creating any shade desired.

However, when mixing to achieve a color different than as packaged by the manufacturer, it is important to remember that a tint with its strong dye load can "overpower" a delicate toner. Because the chemical formulations of tints and toners are comparable and compatible, it is possible to mix the two as long as a *tiny* amount of the tint is used.

When the correct foundation is achieved the color will develop as indicated by the manufacturer. If the finished result appears too flat and ash, the foundation was *over*-lightened. If the finished result appears to have excessive gold or red tones, the foundation was *under*-lightened.

During the application and processing time, toners have a very different color appearance than the final shade. Depending upon the color being used, during this period the toner may appear purple, orange, pink, blue, or a variety of other pastel colors uncommon to hair. This is not cause for panic. As the color oxidizes, it goes through several visual changes. Do a test strand before applying the color to the entire head. This test will insure successful color development and take the worry out of the process.

The experiments in this section are designed to investigate the relationship of achieving the correct level foundation through pre-lightening in order to achieve the hue, level, and saturation desired by the client and intended by the manufacturer. Establishing the correct foundation is the key to all successful toning.

TONING HAIR PRE-LIGHTENED TO STAGE 5

EXPERIMENT INSTRUCTION SHEET

Objectives

To observe and document the color results when toning hair bleached to a stage 5—Gold. This experiment compares the color results when using 10 and 20 volume hydrogen peroxide.

Hair Swatches Needed

6 swatches of hair bleached to stage 5—Gold

Labeling Hair Swatches

- Warm blonde toner/10 volume
- Warm blonde toner/20 volume
- Dark ash blonde toner/10 volume
- Dark ash blonde toner/20 volume
- Neutral toner/10 volume
- Neutral toner/20 volume

Materials Needed

- 20 volume H_2O_2
- 10 volume H_2O_2
- Warm blonde toner
- Dark ash blonde toner
- Neutral toner
- 6 nonmetallic mixing receptacles

Formulation

1. *Swatch #1*—Mix 1 teaspoon of warm blonde toner with appropriate amount of 10 volume hydrogen peroxide in nonmetallic mixing receptacle.
2. *Swatch #2*—Mix 1 teaspoon of warm blonde toner with appropriate amount of 20 volume hydrogen peroxide in nonmetallic mixing receptacle.

3. *Swatch #3*—Mix 1 teaspoon of dark blonde toner with appropriate amount of 10 volume hydrogen peroxide in nonmetallic mixing receptacle.
4. *Swatch #4*—Mix 1 teaspoon of dark ash blonde toner with appropriate amount of 20 volume hydrogen peroxide in nonmetallic mixing receptacle.
5. *Swatch #5*—Mix 1 teaspoon of neutral toner with appropriate amount of 10 volume hydrogen peroxide in nonmetallic mixing receptacle.
6. *Swatch #6*—Mix 1 teaspoon neutral toner with appropriate amount of 20 volume hydrogen peroxide in nonmetallic mixing receptacle.

Procedure

1. Apply each formulation to the appropriately marked swatch.
2. Process at room temperature for 35 minutes.
3. Rinse with cool water, shampoo, and dry.
4. Mount swatches on the *Experiment Results Sheet on page R-159*.
5. Answer the *Review Questions on page R-161*.

TONING HAIR PRE-LIGHTENED TO STAGE 6

EXPERIMENT INSTRUCTION SHEET

Objectives

To observe and document the color results when toning hair bleached to a stage 6—Yellow. This experiment compares the color results when using 10 and 20 volume hydrogen peroxide.

Hair Swatches Needed

6 swatches of hair bleached to stage 6—Yellow

Labeling Hair Swatches

- Beige toner/10 volume
- Beige toner/20 volume
- Ash blonde toner/10 volume
- Ash blonde toner/20 volume
- Golden blonde toner/10 volume
- Golden blonde toner/20 volume

Materials Needed

- 20 volume H_2O_2
- 10 volume H_2O_2
- Beige toner
- Ash blonde toner
- Golden blonde toner
- 6 nonmetallic mixing receptacles

Formulation

1. *Swatch #1*—Mix 1 teaspoon of beige toner with appropriate amount of 10 volume hydrogen peroxide in nonmetallic mixing receptacle.
2. *Swatch #2*—Mix 1 teaspoon of beige toner with appropriate amount of 20 volume hydrogen peroxide in nonmetallic mixing receptacle.
3. *Swatch #3*—Mix 1 teaspoon of ash blonde toner with appropriate amount of 10 volume hydrogen peroxide in nonmetallic mixing receptacle.
4. *Swatch #4*—Mix 1 teaspoon of ash blonde toner with appropriate amount of 20 volume hydrogen peroxide in nonmetallic mixing receptacle.
5. *Swatch #5*—Mix 1 teaspoon of golden blonde toner with appropriate amount of 10 volume hydrogen peroxide in nonmetallic mixing receptacle.
6. *Swatch #6*—Mix 1 teaspoon golden blonde toner with appropriate amount of 20 volume hydrogen peroxide in nonmetallic mixing receptacle.

Procedure

1. Apply each formulation to the appropriately marked swatch.
2. Process at room temperature for 35 minutes.
3. Rinse with cool water, shampoo, and dry.
4. Mount swatches on the *Experiment Results Sheet on page R-163.*
5. Answer the *Review Questions on page R-165.*

TONING HAIR PRE-LIGHTENED TO STAGE 7

EXPERIMENT INSTRUCTION SHEET

Objectives

To observe and document the color results when toning hair bleached to a stage 7—Pale yellow. This experiment compares the color results when using 10 and 20 volume hydrogen peroxide.

Hair Swatches Needed

6 swatches of hair bleached to stage 7—Pale yellow

Labeling Hair Swatches

- White toner/10 volume
- White toner/20 volume
- Silver toner/10 volume
- Silver toner/20 volume
- Platinum toner/10 volume
- Platinum toner/20 volume

Materials Needed

- 20 volume H_2O_2
- 10 volume H_2O_2
- White toner
- Silver toner
- Platinum toner
- 6 nonmetallic mixing receptacles

Formulation

1. *Swatch #1*—Mix 1 teaspoon of white toner with appropriate amount of 10 volume hydrogen peroxide in nonmetallic mixing receptacle.
2. *Swatch #2*—Mix 1 teaspoon of white toner with appropriate amount of 20 volume hydrogen peroxide in nonmetallic mixing receptacle.
3. *Swatch #3*—Mix 1 teaspoon of silver toner with appropriate amount of 10 volume hydrogen peroxide in nonmetallic mixing receptacle.
4. *Swatch #4*—Mix 1 teaspoon of silver toner with appropriate amount of 20 volume hydrogen peroxide in nonmetallic mixing receptacle.
5. *Swatch #5*—Mix 1 teaspoon of platinum toner with appropriate amount of 10 volume hydrogen peroxide in nonmetallic mixing receptacle.
6. *Swatch #6*—Mix 1 teaspoon platinum toner with appropriate amount of 20 volume hydrogen peroxide in nonmetallic mixing receptacle.

Procedure

1. Apply each formulation to the appropriately marked swatch.
2. Process at room temperature for 35 minutes.
3. Rinse with cool water, shampoo, and dry.
4. Mount swatches on the *Experiment Results Sheet on page R-167*.
5. Answer the *Review Questions on page R-169*.

11

Dye Removers

The removal of hair color is sometimes desired for several different reasons. The client may want to change to a lighter hair shade, or the present hair color may have been a mistake. Occasionally color builds up or processes too dark due to an over porous condition of the hair shaft.

Clients rarely want to let the undesirable color grow out naturally. Because the hair only grows ½ inch per month, the client would be left with an unsightly regrowth line for quite a long time. Dye removers are not generally sold for use by nonprofessionals because the process is too complex for the untrained. Therefore, color removing is a professional service that can bring new clients into the salon and convert them to loyal color customers.

Two basic types of products are available to remove artificial pigment from the hair. The first is an oil-base product, which gently removes color build-up or stain that is in the cuticle layer of the hair shaft. The second type is a dye solvent that diffuses and dissolves artificial pigment deposited within the cortex layer of the hair shaft.

OIL-BASE COLOR REMOVERS

The first type of color remover, the oil-base product, only has the power to lift color pigment that has become trapped within the layers of the cuticle. It makes no structural change in the hair shaft or in the pigment (artificial or natural) of the hair. It does no damage to the integrity of the hair.

The oil-base color remover is effectively used to remove temporary color build-up or to lighten slightly a semipermanent or permanent tint that has developed a little too dark. It will not remove a great deal of color or make any drastic change in the level of color.

DYE SOLVENTS

The second type of color remover, the dye solvent, has strong lightening effects on both melanin and artificial pigment. While bleach is the most efficient product to lighten *virgin* hair, it is *not* the best product to use on hair that has previously been darkened or tinted red with an aniline derivative tint. Bleach locks in the golds,

159

oranges, and reds, which occur as artificial hair color progresses through the Seven Stages of Lightening. Because bleach locks in this brassiness, it often becomes impossible to lighten the hair to the desired shade without total destruction of the hair shaft.

A dye solvent is chemically formulated to diffuse and dissolve these artificial color molecules deposited by the aniline derivative tint without locking in brassiness. However, as the dye solvent lightens the artificial color molecules, it also lifts color from the natural pigment or melanin of the hair shaft as well.

Chemical Composition

Sodium hydrosulphite, also known as sodium dithionate, is used in the formulation of dye solvents to deoxidize and reduce the artificial pigment within the cortex. It is a white or grayish white powder that oxidizes in the air. Sodium hydrosulphite also works as a bacterial inhibitor. It is nontoxic and nonallergenic to the skin.

Sodium formaldehyde sulphoxylate and formamidine sulphinic acid are also used effectively to break up the artificial pigment molecules.

Urea peroxide and dry hydrogen peroxide are often found in dye solvents. Both work as oxidizers to diffuse the artificial and natural pigment within the hair shaft. They are drying to the hair and skin but generally cause no allergic reaction.

Polyvinylpyrrolidone, or PVP as it is commonly known, is a solid plastic resin. Used in dye solvents, PVP causes the product to cling to the shaft and helps to create the thickening process that occurs after the product sets for a couple of minutes.

Ethylene glycol monobutyl ether is an ingredient derived from a large class of organic compounds that contain only hydrogen and carbon, such as coal, natural gas, and petroleum. This compound as used in dye solvents also contains glycerin and alcohol. It is alkaline in pH and works as a humectant to retain the moisture within the mixture.

Ammonium carbonate is a solid white alkali derived from ammonium bicarbonate. Ammonium bicarbonate occurs naturally in the urine of alligators. Ammonium carbonate is also used in permanent wave neutralizers.

Ammonia is used in dye solvents in the dry form. It serves the purpose of opening the cuticle and attacking the melanin and artificial pigment within the shaft. It can be very drying to the hair and can even cause breakage if misused.

Carboxymethyl cellulose is a synthetic gum that works as a stabilizer, emulsifier, and foaming agent in dye solvents. It also acts like a barrier agent, which means that it deposits a film that helps to protect the skin from the rest of the ingredients in the dye solvent. Even though carboxymethyl cellulose is believed to cause cancer in animals when ingested, it is used in ice cream, beverages, laxatives, and antacids. Whether or not it is toxic on the skin is unproven at this time.

Safety

Dye solvents, as packaged for professional use, are considered safe. They are nonallergenic and do not require a predisposition test.

Ammonia, ammonium carbonate, sodium formaldehyde sulphoxylate, and formamidine sulphinic acid are also known to be skin irritants that can cause rashes.

However, it is recommended not to sniff the product because the dry powder as well as the fumes from the moist solution as prepared for application can damage the lungs and be irritating to the eyes and mucous membranes. It is especially important to be cautious before and during the mixing as the dry powders of ammonia, PVP, sodium formaldehyde sulfphoxylate, and formamidine sulphinic acid are easily inhaled.

Formulating with Water or Hydrogen Peroxide

Some dye solvents may be mixed only with hydrogen peroxide. Others have the option of being mixed with water to create a milder color remover. Check the individual manufacturer's recommended directions.

Formulating with hydrogen peroxide creates a product that is quite strong and generally will remove any artificial pigment with the exception of the polymer colors. The option of using water to create a gentler product is often desirable but can lead to inconsistent results.

The reason for this is that calcium and magnesium are two metals found in tap water. These metals cause quick release of the extra oxygen atom in peroxide, which is the key ingredient in most prepared dye solvents. The amount of metal in tap water is unknown to the colorist and can vary from day to day. Therefore, the water formula may create unreliable results unless de-ionized, distilled, or purified water is used.

ACTION OF DYE SOLVENT

EXPERIMENT INSTRUCTION SHEET

Objectives

To observe and document the action and decolorizing results of dye solvent use. To gain experience mixing and formulating a dye solvent.

Hair Swatches Needed

Swatches should be from same head cutting:

- 2 swatches of tinted level 1—Black hair
- 2 swatches of tinted level 4—Light brown hair

Labeling Hair Swatches

Label one brown and one black swatch to indicate that a water formula will be used on them. Label the other brown and black swatch to indicate that a hydrogen peroxide formula will be used on them.

Materials Needed

- 20 volume hydrogen peroxide
- Distilled water

- Dye solvent (one that can be mixed with both water and hydrogen peroxide)
- Waxed paper

Procedure

1. Arrange labeled hair swatches on waxed paper in two groups. Place together the two swatches to which the H_2O_2 formula will be applied. Place together the two swatches on which the H_2O formula will be used.
2. Mix a small amount of dye solvent with H_2O according to the manufacturer's recommended directions.
3. Allow both formulas to set a couple of minutes to thicken. Stir gently.
4. Thoroughly saturate one tinted brown swatch and one tinted black swatch with the H_2O_2 mixture.
5. Thoroughly saturate one tinted brown swatch and one tinted black swatch with the H_2O mixture.
6. Process at room temperature for 45 minutes.
7. Rinse, shampoo, dry.
8. Mount swatches on the *Experiment Results Sheet on page R-171.*
9. Answer *Review Questions on page R-173.*

TINTING AFTER THE USE OF A DYE SOLVENT

The use of a dye solvent does not, as a general rule, create a finished result. Double application hair coloring is almost always necessary. The color resulting from the use of a dye solvent is rarely even and is usually red, orange, or gold.

After the artificial pigment has been successfully removed, there are several options available to achieve a finished product. The hair may now be tinted, toned, or bleached to achieve the desired shade. However, before continuing, analyze the hair to decide whether or not the hair and scalp can withstand another chemical application.

If possible, condition the hair and wait 24 hours before proceeding. Within this time span, the sebaceous glands will secrete natural oils that help protect the scalp from chemical burns. It also gives the hair time to return to its natural pH and for the pores of the scalp to return to normal. This 24-hour grace period is a safety precaution, but it is not mandatory. If the hair is treated properly, the color service usually can be completed in one day.

Regardless of whether the new color is applied immediately, or 24 hours later, the hair shaft will have a new porosity factor to consider. Remember, the hair has already been treated at least twice with chemicals. Application of either a tint or dye solvent causes the hair to become more porous. In this case, both chemicals have been applied to the hair.

A tint applied to porous hair will create a darker hue than if it is applied to nonporous hair. Therefore, when selecting the tint to be applied after use of a dye solvent, select a hue that is at least one level lighter than would be used on hair of normal porosity.

Hair that is completely depleted may have the opposite color problem. Occasionally, the color applied after the use of the dye solvent will *not* process as dark as the desired shade and leaves the hair with a "gun metal gray" tone. This indicates that the hair is so over-porous that there are insufficient protein bonds and natural melanin left within the cortex for the artificial pigment to attach to. The lighter than expected color result is a real danger sign. Hair that is this porous is very fragile and may be close to the breaking point.

In both instances, the color will process cooler than it would on undamaged hair. The Artist's Concept of the Laws of Color must be used to add the missing foundation warmth when formulating the tint to be used after a dye solvent.

Because of these factors, it is often desirable to include the use of a filler with this procedure. Refer to the section on fillers for the three standard methods of use to decide which is appropriate for the amount of porosity in each individual case.

Formulations incorporating the theory of low volume peroxide for a milder solution that deposits without lifting are often used in tinting hair that has been treated with a dye remover.

Regardless of the chosen method, a test strand is a *must* before beginning this service. The condition of the hair, the reduced moisture content, the elasticity, and increased porosity set the stage for unpredictable color results. Each case is different!

**TINTING AFTER DYE REMOVAL
20 VOLUME FORMULATION**

EXPERIMENT INSTRUCTION SHEET

Objectives

To gain experience tinting hair that has undergone dye removal. To observe and document the color results due to the porosity created by the dye solvent.

Hair Swatches Needed

4 swatches of previously tinted hair from the same head cutting

Labeling Hair Swatches

Label swatches as follows:

- Level 8—Light blonde
- Level 6—Dark blonde
- Level 4—Light brown
- Level 2—Dark brown

Materials Needed

- 20 volume hydrogen peroxide
- Dye solvent
- Level 8—Light blonde tint

- Level 6—Dark blonde tint
- Level 4—Light brown tint
- Level 2—Dark brown tint

Dye Solvent Formulation

1. Read manufacturer's recommended directions. Using the formula that requires hydrogen peroxide, measure ½ the amount necessary for a complete application.
2. Allow to set a moment to thicken. Stir gently.
3. Thoroughly saturate all swatches.
4. Process at room temperature for 45 minutes.
5. Rinse, shampoo, and dry.

Tint Procedure

1. Select one tint from each of the color levels as indicated on the labels of the swatches.
2. Mix 1 teaspoon of each tint with the appropriate amount of 20 volume hydrogen peroxide.
3. Thoroughly saturate the appropriately labeled hair swatches.
4. Process at room temperature for 35 minutes.
5. Rinse, shampoo, and dry.
6. Mount swatches on the *Experiment Results Sheet on page R-175.*
7. Answer *Review Questions on page R-177.*

TINTING AFTER DYE REMOVAL
10 VOLUME FORMULATION

EXPERIMENT INSTRUCTION SHEET

Objectives

To gain experience tinting hair that has undergone dye removal. To observe and document the color results due to the porosity created by the dye solvent.

Hair Swatches Needed

4 swatches of previously tinted hair from the same head cutting

Labeling Hair Swatches

Label swatches as follows:

- Level 8—Light blonde
- Level 6—Dark blonde
- Level 4—Light brown
- Level 2—Dark brown

Materials Needed

- 10 and 20 volume hydrogen peroxide
- Dye solvent
- Level 8—Light blonde tint
- Level 6—Dark blonde tint
- Level 4—Light brown tint
- Level 2—Dark brown tint

Dye Solvent Formulation

1. Read manufacturer's recommended directions. Using the formula that requires 20 volume hydrogen peroxide, measure ½ the amount necessary for a complete application.
2. Allow to set a moment to thicken. Stir gently.
3. Thoroughly saturate all swatches.
4. Process at room temperature for 45 minutes.
5. Rinse, shampoo, and dry.

Tint Procedure

1. Select one tint from each of the color levels as indicated on the labels of the swatches.
2. Mix 1 teaspoon of each tint with the appropriate amount of 10 volume hydrogen peroxide.
3. Thoroughly saturate the appropriately labeled hair swatches.
4. Process at room temperature for 35 minutes.
5. Rinse, shampoo, and dry.
6. Mount swatches on the *Experiment Results Sheet on page R-179*.
7. Answer *Review Questions on page R-181*.

> ### TINTING AFTER DYE REMOVAL
> ### FILLER FORMULATION
>
> *EXPERIMENT INSTRUCTION SHEET*

Objectives

To gain experience utilizing a filler when tinting hair that has undergone dye removal. To observe and document the color results due to the porosity created by the dye solvent.

Hair Swatches Needed

4 swatches of previously tinted hair from the same head cutting

Labeling Hair Swatches

Label swatches as follows:

- Level 8—Light blonde
- Level 6—Dark blonde
- Level 4—Light brown
- Level 2—Dark brown

Materials Needed

- 20 volume hydrogen peroxide
- Dye solvent
- Level 8—Light blonde tint
- Level 6—Dark blonde tint
- Level 4—Light brown tint
- Level 2—Dark brown tint
- Yellow filler
- Gold filler
- Orange filler
- Red filler

Dye Solvent Formulation

1. Read manufacturer's recommended directions. Using the formula that requires hydrogen peroxide, measure ½ the amount necessary for a complete application.

2. Allow to set a moment to thicken. Stir gently.
3. Thoroughly saturate all swatches.
4. Process at room temperature for 45 minutes.
5. Rinse, shampoo, and dry.

Tint Procedure

1. Select one tint from each of the color levels as indicated on the labels of the swatches.
2. Mix 1 teaspoon of each tint with the appropriate amount of 20 volume hydrogen peroxide.

Addition of Filler

1. Add 1 teaspoon yellow filler to light blonde tint.
2. Add 1 teaspoon gold filler to dark blonde tint.
3. Add 1 teaspoon orange filler to light brown tint.
4. Add 1 teaspoon red filler to dark brown tint.

Application

1. Thoroughly saturate appropriately labeled hair swatches.
2. Process at room temperature for 35 minutes.
3. Rinse, shampoo, and dry.
4. Mount swatches on the *Experiment Results Sheet on page R-183.*
5. Answer *Review Questions on page R-185.*

Glossary

(We include this glossary with the intention of helping to standardize the language for hair color. It has been prepared and authorized by the International Haircolor Exchange, an organization interested in furthering hair color education.)

accelerator: (See *activator*)

accent color: A concentrated color product that can be added to permanent, semi-permanent or temporary haircolor to intensify or tone down the color. Another word for concentrate.

acid: An aqueous (water based) solution having a pH less than 7.0 on the pH scale.

activator: An additive used to quicken the action or progress of a chemical. Another word for booster, accelerator, protenator or catalyst.

alkaline: An aqueous (water based) solution having a pH greater than 7.0 on the pH scale. The opposite of acid.

allergy: A reaction due to extreme sensitivity to certain foods or chemicals.

allergy test: A test to determine the possibility or degree of sensitivity, also known as a patch test, predisposition test or skin test.

amino acids: The group of molecules which the body uses to synthesize protein. There are some 22 different amino acids found in living protein that serve as units of structure in protein.

ammonia: A colorless pungent gas composed of hydrogen and nitrogen; in water solution it is called ammonia water. Used in haircolor to swell the cuticle. When mixed with hydrogen peroxide, activates the oxidation process on melanin and allows the melanin to decolorize.

ammonium hydroxide: An alkali solution of ammonia in water, commonly used in the manufacture of permanent haircolor, lightener preparations, and hair relaxers.

analysis (hair): An examination of the hair to determine its condition and natural color. (See *consultation, condition*)

aqueous: Descriptive term for water solution or any medium that is largely composed of water.

ash: A tone or shade dominated by greens, blues, violets or grays. May be used to counteract unwanted warm tones.

base (alkali): (See *pH; alkaline*)

base color: (See *color base*)

bleeding: Seepage of tint/lightener from foil or cap due to improper application.

blending: A merging of one tint or tone with another.

blonding: A term applied to lightening the hair.

bonds: The means by which atoms are joined together to make molecules.

booster: (See *activator*)

brassy tone: Red, orange or gold tones in the hair.

breakage: A condition in which hair splits and breaks off.

build-up: Repeated coatings on the hair shaft.

catalyst: A substance used to alter the speed of a chemical reaction.

caustic: Strongly alkaline materials. At very high pH levels, can burn or destroy protein or tissue by chemical action.

certified color: A color which meets certain standards for purity and is certified by the FDA.

cetyl alcohol: Fatty alcohol used as an emollient. It is also used as a stabilizer for emulsion systems and in haircolor and cream developer as a thickener.

chelating stabilizer: A molecule that binds metal ions and renders them inactive.

chemical change: Alteration in the chemical composition of a substance.

citric acid: Organic acid derived from citrus fruits and used for pH adjustment. Primarily used to adjust the acid-alkali balance. Has some antioxidant and preservative qualities. Used medicinally as a mild astringent.

coating: Residue left on the outside of the hair shaft.

color: Visual sensation caused by light.

color additive: (See *accent color*)

color base: The combination of dyes which make up the tonal foundation of a specific haircolor.

color lift: The amount of change natural or artificial pigment undergoes when lightened by a substance.

color mixing: Combining two or more shades together for a custom color.

color refresher: 1. Color applied to midshaft and ends to give a more uniform color appearance to the hair. 2. Color applied by a shampoo-in method to enhance the natural color. Also called color wash, color enhancer.

color remover: A product designed to remove artificial pigment from the hair.

color test: The process of removing product from a hair strand to monitor the progress of color development during tinting or lightening.

color wheel: The arrangement of primary and secondary and tertiary colors in the order of their relationships to each other. A tool for formulating.

complementary colors: A primary and secondary color positioned opposite each other on the color wheel. When these two colors are combined, they create a neutral color. Combinations are as follows: Blue/Orange, Red/Green, Yellow/Violet.

concentrate: (See *accent color*)

condition: The existing state of the hair; elasticity, strength, texture, porosity and evidence of previous treatments.

consultation: Verbal communication with a client to determine desired result. [See *analysis (hair)*]

contributing pigment: The current level and tone of the hair: Refers to both natural contributing pigment and decolorized (or lightened) contributing pigment. (See *undertone*)

cool tones: (See *ash*)

corrective coloring: The process of correcting an undesirable color.

cortex: The second layer of hair. A fibrous protein core of the hair fiber, containing melanin pigment.

coverage: Reference to the ability of a color product to color gray, white or other colors of hair.

cuticle: The translucent protein outer layer of the hair fiber.

cysteic acid: A chemical substance, in the hair fiber, produced by the interaction of hydrogen peroxide on the disulfide bond (cystine).

cystine: The disulfide amino acid which joins protein chains together.

D & C colors: Colors selected from a certified list approved by the Food and Drug Administration for use in drug and cosmetic products.

decolorize: A chemical process involving the lightening of the natural color pigment or artificial color from the hair.

degree: Term used to describe various units of measurement.

dense: Thick, compact or crowded.

deposit: Describes the color product in terms of its ability to add color pigment to the hair. Color added equals deposit.

deposit only color: A category of color products between permanent and semi-permanent colors. Formulated to only deposit color, not lift. They contain oxidation dyes and utilize low volume developer.

depth: The lightness or darkness of a specific haircolor. (See *value, level*)

developer: An oxidizing agent, usually hydrogen peroxide, that reacts chemically with coloring material to develop color molecules and create a change in natural hair color.

development time (oxidation period): The time required for a permanent color or lightener to completely develop.

diffused: Broken down, scattered; not limited to one spot.

direct dye: A pre-formed color which dyes the fiber directly without the need for oxidation.

discoloration: The development of undesired shades through chemical reaction.

double process: A technique requiring two separate procedures in which the hair is decolorized or pre-lightened with a lightener before the depositing color is applied.

drab: Term used to describe haircolor shades containing no red or gold. (See *ash; dull*)

drabber: Concentrated color, used to reduce red or gold highlights.

dull: A word used to describe hair or haircolor without sheen.

dye: Artificial pigment.

dye intermediate: A material which develops into color only after reaction with developer (hydrogen peroxide). Also known as oxidation dyes.

dye solvents or dye remover: (See *color remover*)

dye stock: (See *color base*)

elasticity: The ability of the hair to stretch and return to normal.

enzyme: A protein molecule found in living cells which initiates a chemical process.

fade: To lose color through exposure to the elements or other factors.

fillers: 1. Color product used as a color refresher or to fill damaged hair in preparation for haircoloring. 2. Any liquid-like substance to help fill a void. (See *color refresher*)

formulas: Mixtures of two or more ingredients.

formulate: The art of mixing to create a blend or balance of two or more ingredients.

gray hair: Hair with decreasing amounts of natural pigment. Hair with no natural pigment is actually white. White hairs look gray when mingled with the still pigmented hair.

hair: A slender threadlike outgrowth of the skin of the head and body.

hair root: That part of the hair contained within the follicle, below the surface of the scalp.

hair shaft: Visible part of each strand of hair. It is made up of an outer layer called the cuticle, an innermost layer called medulla and an in-between layer called the cortex. The cortex layer is where color changes are made.

hard water: Water which contains minerals and metallic salts as impurities.

henna: A plant extracted coloring which produces bright shades of red. The active ingredient is lawsone. Henna permanently colors the hair by coating and penetrating the hair shaft. (See *progressive dye*)

high lift tinting: A single process color with a higher degree of lightening action and a minimal amount of color deposit.

highlighting: The introduction of a lighter color in small selected sections to increase lightness of hair. Generally not strongly contrasting from the natural color.

hydrogen peroxide: An oxidizing chemical made up of 2 parts hydrogen, 2 parts oxygen (H_2O_2) used to aid the processing of permanent haircolor and lighteners. Also referred to as a developer, available in liquid or cream.

level: A unit of measurement, used to evaluate the lightness or darkness of a color, excluding tone.

level system: In haircoloring, a system colorists use to analyze the lightness or darkness of a haircolor.

lift: The lightening action of a haircolor or lightening product on the hair's natural pigment.

lightener: The chemical compound which lightens the hair by dispersing, dissolving and decolorizing the natural hair pigment. (See *pre-lighten*)

lightening: (See *decolorize*)

line of demarcation: An obvious difference between two colors on the hair shaft.

litmus paper: A chemically-treated paper used to test the acidity or alkalinity of products.

medulla: The center structure of the hair shaft. Little is known about its actual function.

melanin: The tiny grains of pigment in the hair cortex which create natural hair color.

melanocytes: Cells in the hair bulb that manufacture melanin.

melanoprotein: The protein coating of a melanosome.

melanosome: Protein-coated granule containing melanin.

metallic dyes: Soluble metal salts such as lead, silver, and bismuth which produce colors on the hair fiber by progressive build-up and exposure to air.

modifier: A chemical found as an ingredient in permanent haircolors. Its function is to alter the dye intermediates.

molecule: Two or more atoms chemically joined together; the smallest part of a compound.

neutral: 1. A color balanced between warm and cool, which does not reflect a highlight of any primary or secondary color. 2. Also refers to a pH of 7.

neutralization: The process that counter-balances or cancels the action of an agent or color.

neutralize: Render neutral; counter-balance of action or influence. (See *neutral*)

new growth: The part of the hair shaft which is between previously chemically treated hair and the scalp.

nonalkaline: (See *acid*)

off the scalp lightener: Generally a stronger lightener usually in powder form, not to be used directly on the scalp.

on the scalp lightener: A liquid, cream or gel form of lightener that can be used directly on the scalp.

opaque: Allowing no light to shine through.

outgrowth (See *new growth*)

over-lap: Occurs when the application of color or lightener goes beyond the line of demarcation.

over-porosity: The condition where hair reaches an undesirable stage of porosity requiring correction.

oxidation: 1. The reaction of dye intermediates with hydrogen peroxide found in haircoloring developers. 2. The interaction of hydrogen peroxide on the natural pigment.

oxidative hair color: A product containing oxidation dyes which require hydrogen peroxide to develop the permanent color.

para tint: A tint made from oxidation dyes.

para-phenylenediamine: An oxidation dye used in most permanent haircolors, often abbreviated as P.P.D.

patch test: A test required by the Food and Drug Act. Made by applying a small amount of the haircoloring preparation to the skin of the arm or behind the ear to determine possible allergies (Hypersensitivity). Also called pre-disposition or skin test.

penetrating color: Color which enters or penetrates the cortex or second layer of the hair shaft.

permanent color: 1. Haircolor products which do not wash out by shampooing. 2. A category of haircolor products mixed with developer that create a lasting color change.

peroxide: (See *hydrogen peroxide*)

peroxide residue: Traces of peroxide left in the hair after treatment with lightener or tint.

persulfate: In haircoloring, a chemical ingredient commonly used in activators. It increases the speed of the decolorization process. (See *activator*)

pH: The quantity which expresses the acid/alkali balance. A pH of 7 is the neutral value for pure water. Any pH below 7 is acidic; any pH above 7 is alkaline. The skin is mildly acidic and generally in the pH 4.5 to 5.5 range.

pH scale: A numerical scale from 0 (very acid) to 14 (very alkaline), used to describe the degree of acidity or alkalinity.

pigment: Any substance or matter used as coloring: natural or artificial haircolor.

porosity: Ability of the hair to absorb water or other liquids.

powder lightener: (See *off the scalp lightener*)

pre-bleaching: (See *pre-lighten*)

pre-disposition test: (See *patch test*)

pre-lighten: Generally the first step of double process haircoloring. To lift or lighten the natural pigment. (See *decolorize*)

pre-soften: The process of treating gray or very resistant hair to allow for better penetration of color.

primary colors: Pigments or colors that are fundamental and cannot be made by mixing colors together. Red, yellow and blue are the primary colors.

prism: A transparent glass or crystal solid which breaks up white light into its component colors, the spectrum.

processing time: The time required for the chemical treatment to react on the hair.

progressive dyes or progressive dye system: 1. A coloring system which produces increased absorption with each application. 2. Color products that deepen or increase absorption over a period of time during processing.

regrowth: (See *new growth*)

resistant hair: Hair which is difficult to penetrate with moisture or chemical solutions.

retouch: Application of color or lightening mixture to new growth of hair.

salt and pepper: The descriptive term for a mixture of dark and gray or white hair.

secondary color: Colors made by combining two primary colors in equal proportion: Green, Orange and Violet are secondary colors.

semi-permanent hair coloring: Hair coloring that lasts through several shampoos. It penetrates the hair shaft and stains the cuticle layer, slowly diffusing out with each shampoo.

sensitivity: A skin highly reactive to the presence of a specific chemical. Skin reddens or becomes irritated shortly after application of the chemical. On removal of the chemical, the reaction subsides.

shade: 1. A term used to describe a specific color. 2. The visible difference between two colors.

sheen: The ability of the hair to shine, gleam, or reflect light.

single process color: Refers to an oxidative tint solution that lifts or lightens while also depositing color in one application. (See *oxidative hair color*)

softening agent: A mild alkaline product applied prior to the color treatment, to increase porosity, swell the cuticle layer of the hair and increase color absorption. Tint that has not been mixed with developer is frequently used. (See *pre-soften*)

solution: A blended mixture of solid, liquid or gaseous substances in a liquid medium.

solvent: Carrier liquid in which other components may be dissolved.

specialist: One who concentrates on only one part or branch of a subject or profession.

spectrum: The series of colored bands diffracted and arranged in the order of their wavelengths by the passage of white light through a prism. Shading continuously from red (produced by the longest wave visible) to violet (produced by the shortest): Red, Orange, Yellow, Green, Blue, Indigo and Violet.

spot lightening: Color correcting using a lightening mixture to lighten darker areas.

stabilizer: General name for ingredient which prolongs lifetime, appearance and performance of a product.

stage: A term used to describe a visible color change that natural hair color goes through while being lightened.

stain remover: Chemical used to remove tint stains from skin.

strand test: Test given before treatment to determine development time, color result and the ability of the hair to withstand the effects of chemicals.

stripping: (See *color remover*)

surfactant: A short way of saying Surface Active Agent. A molecule which is composed of an oil-loving (oleophillic) part and a water-loving (hydrophilic) part. They act as a bridge to allow oil and water to mix. Wetting agents, emulsifiers, cleansers, solubilizers, dispersing aids and thickeners are usually surfactants.

tablespoon: 1/2 of an ounce. 3 teaspoons.

teaspoon: 1/6 of an ounce. 1/3 of a tablespoon.

temporary coloring or temporary rinses: Color made from pre-formed dyes which are applied to the hair, but are readily removed with shampoo.

terminology: The special words or terms used in science, art or business.

tertiary colors: The mixture of a primary and an adjacent secondary color on the color wheel. Red-orange, Yellow-orange, Yellow-green, Blue-green, Blue-violet, Red-violet. Also referred to as intermediary colors.

texture, hair: The diameter of an individual hair strand. Termed: coarse, medium or fine.

tint: Permanent oxidizing haircolor product having the ability to lift and deposit color in the same process.

tint back: To return hair back to its original or natural color.

tone: A term used to describe the warmth or coolness in color.

toner: A pastel color to be used after pre-lightening.

toning: Adding color to modify the end result.

touch-up: (See *retouch*)

translucent: The property of letting diffused light pass through.

tyrosine: The amino acid (tyrosine) which reacts together with the enzyme (tyrosinase) to form the hair's natural melanin.

tyrosinase: The enzyme (tyrosinase) which reacts together with the amino acid (tyrosine) to form the hair's natural melanin.

undertone: The underlying color that emerges during the lifting process of melanin, that contributes to the end result. When lightening hair, a residual warmth in tone always occurs.

urea peroxide: A peroxide compound occasionally used in haircolor. When added to an alkaline color mixture, it releases oxygen.

value: (See *level; depth*)

vegetable color: A color derived from plant sources.

virgin hair: Natural hair that has not undergone any chemical or physical abuse.

viscosity: A term referring to the thickness of the solution.

volume: The concentration of hydrogen peroxide in water solution. Expressed as volumes of oxygen liberated per volume of solution. 20 volume peroxide would thus liberate 20 pints of oxygen gas for each pint of solution.

warm: Containing red, orange, yellow or gold tones.

Bibliography

Adrosko, Rita. *Natural Dyes in the United States*. Washington, D.C.: Smithsonian Institution Press, 1968.

Allen, R.L.M. Imperial Chemical Industries Limited, *Colour Chemistry*. New York: Meredith Corporation, 1971.

Birren, Faber. *Light, Color and Environment*. New York: Van Nostrand Reinhold Company, 1969.

Brandley, Franklyn M. *Color*. New York: Thomas Y. Crowell Company, 1978.

Burnham, Robert W., Hanes, Randall M., Bartleson, C. James. *COLOR: A Guide to Basic Facts and Concepts*. New York: John Wiley and Sons, Inc., 1963.

Collier's Encyclopedia. *Dyes and Dyeing*. London: P.F. Collier Inc., 1981, Vol. 8, pp. 456-457.

Corbet, John F., vice president, technology, Clairol. "Melanin—The Source of Natural Hair Color." Manuscript scheduled for future publication in the *Clairol Salon Professional Magazine*.

Corbet, John F., vice president, technology, Clairol. "The Bleaching of Melanin." Manuscript scheduled for future publication in the *Clairol Salon Professional Magazine*.

Corbet, John F., vice president, technology, Clairol. Personal communication of December 11, 1987.

Davis, Donald A. "Hair Care Market; ever more segmentation." *Drug and Cosmetic Industry*, Vol. 140, April 1987, pp. 32-38.

Demachy, Alain. *Interior Architecture and Decoration*. New York: William Morrow and Company, Inc., 1974.

DeNavarre, Maison G., Ph.C, B.S., M.S. *The Chemistry and Manufacture of Cosmetics*, 2nd edition. New Jersey: D. Van Nostrand Company, Incorporated, 1962.

Editors of Consumer Reports Books. *The Medicine Show*. New York: Pantheon Books, 1980.

Encyclopedia Americana. *Color*. Connecticut: Grolier Incorporated, 1985, Vol. 7, pp. 305-315.

Food and Drug Administration. *Requirements of Laws and Regulations Enforced by the U.S. Food and Drug Administration*, U.S. Department of Health and Human Services, Washington, D.C., 78 pages plus additional xeroxed sheets.

Harry, Ralph G., edited by George Godwin. *Harry's Cosmeticology*. New York: Chemical Publishing Company, Incorporated, 1982.

Healy, Mary. "Ethnic Coloring Techniques." *National Beauty School Journal,* Vol. 39, No. 7, July 1987, pp. 6-7.

Howard, George M., revised by Poucher, W.A. *Perfumes, Cosmetics and Soaps*. New York: John Wiley and Sons, 1987.

Libby, William Charles. *Color and the Structural Sense*. New Jersey: Prentice-Hall, Inc., 1974.

Mayer, Ralph. *The Painter's Craft*. New York: The Viking Press, 1975.

McGraw Hill Encyclopedia of Science and Technology. *Color*. New York: McGraw Hill Book Company, 1987, pp. 164-176.

Meyer, W. and Blood, Ida. *The Cosmetiste*. Illinois: W.M. Meyer Co., 1928.

Milady's Standard Textbook of Cosmetology. New York: Milady Publishing Company, 1991.

1987 Modern's Market Guide. *Color*. Illinois: Vance Publishing Guide, pp. 21-26, 256-280.

1986 Modern's Market Guide. *Color*. Illinois: Vance Publishing Guide, pp. 29-32.

1985 Modern's Market Guide. *Color*. Illinois: Vance Publishing Guide, pp. 39-44, 56-57.

1984 Modern's Market Guide. *Color*. Illinois: Vance Publishing Guide, pp. 39, 43, 44, 148.

1983 Modern's Market Guide. *Color*. Illinois: Vance Publishing Guide, pp. 35, 36, 38, 48.

1982 Modern's Market Guide. *Color*. Illinois: Vance Publishing Guide, pp. 33-36.

1981 Modern's Market Guide. *Color*. Illinois: Vance Publishing Guide, pp. 21-27, 78.

National Cancer Institute (U.S.). Bioassay of testing for possible carcinogenicity, Carcinogenesis Testing Program, National Cancer Institute, National Institute of Health, and National Toxicology Program, Bethesda, Maryland, 1980.

National Toxicology Program. Technical report series on toxicology and carcinogenesis studies of HC Blue no. 2:-2.2 (4-92-hydroxyethylamino)bis(ethanol), Public Health Department, 1987.

National Toxicology Program. National Technical Information Service report, Case #33229-34-4, Testing on rats and mice, August 1986.

Pavey, Donald. *Color*. California: Marshall Editions Limited, The Knapp Press, 1980.

Pellew, Donald, Professor of Chemistry. *Dyes and Dyeing*. New York: Robert M. McBride and Company, 1921.

Powitt, A.H., B.Sc., A.S.T.C. *Hair Structure and Chemistry Simplified*. New York: Milady Publishing Company, 1977.

Rinzler, Carol Ann. *Cosmetics: What the Ads Don't Tell You*. New York: Thomas Y. Crowell Company, 1987.

Roux Laboratories, Inc. *Materials Safety Sheet: Semipermanent Hair Dyes*, July 16, 1985.

Roux Laboratories, Inc. *Materials Safety Sheet: Semipermanent Hair Dye—Part II Activator*, September 19, 1986.

Roux Laboratories, Inc. *Materials Safety Sheet: Temporary Dyes*, July 16, 1985.

Roux Laboratories, Inc. *Materials Safety Sheet: Permanent Hair Dyes*, July 16, 1985.

Science Action Coalition. *Consumer's Guide to Cosmetics*. New York: Anchor Press/ Doubleday, 1980.

Scott, Callahan, Faulkner, Jenkins, Nunz, Ponce-Hantz and Sterner. *Prentice-Hall Textbook of Cosmetology*. New Jersey: Prentice-Hall, Inc.

Spencer, Patricia A., Associate Professor of Cosmetology. "KINETIC MOLECULAR THEORY: Where Does the Color Go?" *National Beauty School Journal*, Vol. 39, No. 7, July 1987, p. 25.

Spencer, Patricia A., Associate Professor of Cosmetology. "Teaching Sales Techniques." *National Beauty School Journal*, Vol. 39, No. 10, October 1987, pp. 10,11, 28.

Stabile, Toni. *Everything You Wanted to Know About Cosmetics*. New York: Dodd, Mead, and Company, 1984.

Subcommittee on Oversight and Investigation of Committee on Interstate and Foreign Commerce. Hearings on safety of hair dyes and cosmetic products, House of Representatives, Ninety-sixth Congress, first session, U.S. Government Printing Office, 1980.

Swaton, Jr., J. Norman. *Chemistry: A Programmed Text*. Intron Inc., 1976.

Tenerelli, Mary Jane. "The Development of Cosmetology Hair Coloring." *National Beauty School Journal*, Vol. 37, No. 4, April 1985, pp. 14-15.

U.S. Department of Health. *Suspected Carcinogens: A Subfile of the Registry of Toxic Effects of Chemical Substances*, Center for Disease Control.

United States Congressional Report. *Lack of Authority Hampers Attempts to Increase Cosmetic Safety*, Washington, D.C., 1986.

"Use Color to Bring Life to Your Surroundings." The Press-Enterprise, Riverside, California, October 10, 1987.

Viera, James W. *Guide to Professional Hair Coloring and Hair Care*. New York: L'Oreal, 1979.

Winter, Ruth. *Dictionary of Cosmetic Ingredients*. New York: Crown Publishers, Inc., 1984.

The World Book Encyclopedia. *Color*. Chicago: World Book Incorporated, 1987, Vol. 4, pp. 660-667.

Zotos Product Science. New York: Zotos International, Inc., 1987.

Index

Experiment Results Sheets

and

Review Questions

LEVEL 8—SEMIPERMANENT COLOR RESULTS COMPARISON
EXPERIMENT RESULTS SHEET

**Natural Level
8-9**

**Natural Level
5-6**

**Natural Level
2-3**

**Natural
Salt and Pepper**

Color Name and Number _____

Manufacturer _____

Formulation _____

Timing _____

Comments _____

_____

LEVEL 8—SEMIPERMANENT COLOR RESULTS COMPARISON

REVIEW QUESTIONS

1. Compare the color results achieved on the four different natural colors.

2. Did the blonde semipermanent color lighten the dark hair?

   Why or why not?

3. List three advantages of using semipermanent color.

4. Is a predisposition test required before semipermanent color application?

5. Which ingredients in semipermanent colors cause them to penetrate the hair shaft?

LEVEL 5-6—AUBURN SEMIPERMANENT COLOR RESULTS COMPARISON

EXPERIMENT RESULTS SHEET

**Natural Level
8-9**

**Natural Level
5-6**

**Natural Level
2-3**

**Natural
Salt and Pepper**

Color Name and Number _____

Manufacturer _____

Formulation _____

Timing _____

Comments _____

_____

LEVEL 5-6—AUBURN SEMIPERMANENT COLOR RESULTS COMPARISON

REVIEW QUESTIONS

1. Compare the color results achieved on the four different natural colors.

2. Is auburn an appropriate color for use on all natural colors of hair?

3. Do semipermanent colors make a chemical or structural change in the hair shaft?

4. Does the fact that the client had auburn hair in youth guarantee that the color will always be flattering?

   Why?

5. What is the approximate pH range of semipermanent colors?

LEVEL 3—SEMIPERMANENT COLOR RESULTS COMPARISON

EXPERIMENT RESULTS SHEET

**Natural Level
8-9**

**Natural Level
5-6**

**Natural Level
2-3**

**Natural
Salt and Pepper**

Color Name and Number _____

Manufacturer _____

Formulation _____

Timing _____

Comments _____

_____

LEVEL 3—SEMIPERMANENT COLOR RESULTS COMPARISON

REVIEW QUESTIONS

1. Compare the color results achieved on the four different natural colors.

2. Did the brown semipermanent color lighten the dark hair?

   Why or why not?

3. Approximately how long will this type of coloring remain on the hair?

4. Describe the problems that can occur when using a brown semipermanent color.

5. What is the key ingredient in the composition of the activator used with many semipermanent colors?

LEVEL 1—SEMIPERMANENT COLOR RESULTS COMPARISON

EXPERIMENT RESULTS SHEET

**Natural Level
8-9**

**Natural Level
5-6**

**Natural Level
2-3**

**Natural
Salt and Pepper**

Color Name and Number _____

Manufacturer _____

Formulation_____

Timing_____

Comments _____

_____

LEVEL 1—SEMIPERMANENT COLOR RESULTS COMPARISON

REVIEW QUESTIONS

1. Compare the color results on the four different natural colors.

2. Is black an appropriate color for use on all natural colors of hair?

3. What types of pigments are used in semipermanent colors?

4. Does the fact that the client had black hair in youth guarantee that the color will always be flattering?

    Why?

5. What is the purpose of the after-rinse provided with some semipermanent colors?

SEMIPERMANENT HAIR COLOR BRAND COMPARISON

EXPERIMENT RESULTS SHEET

Level 7-8

Manufacturer _____   Manufacturer _____

Color _____   Color _____

Formulation _____   Formulation _____

Level 4-5

Manufacturer _____   Manufacturer _____

Color _____   Color _____

Formulation _____   Formulation _____

Level 1-2

Manufacturer _____   Manufacturer _____

Color _____   Color _____

Formulation _____   Formulation _____

SEMIPERMANENT HAIR COLOR BRAND COMPARISON

REVIEW QUESTIONS

1. Do these semipermanent colors coat or penetrate the hair shaft? What size are the pigment molecules in this type of color?

2. Why are they called "semipermanent"?

3. List the main uses of this classification of color.

4. How do the colors of the two different brands compare?

5. Did the colors you selected achieve the tone and depth that you expected?

   Explain your conclusions.

NATURAL POLYMER COLORS

EXPERIMENT RESULTS SHEET

Clear

| **Level 7 or 8** | **Level 4 or 5** | **Level 2 or 3** |

Medium Gold

| **Level 7 or 8** | **Level 4 or 5** | **Level 2 or 3** |

Soft Brown

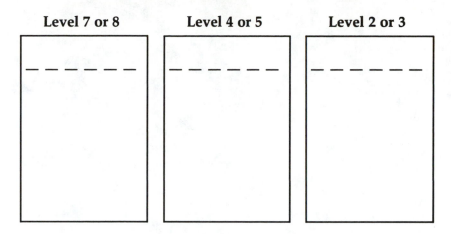

Level 7 or 8 **Level 4 or 5** **Level 2 or 3**

Natural Auburn

Level 7 or 8 **Level 4 or 5** **Level 2 or 3**

NATURAL POLYMER COLOR COMPARISON

REVIEW QUESTIONS

1. Describe two uses for clear polymer colors.

2. What is the most important step of professional color selection?

3. What type of dyes are used in polymer colors?

4. Define polymer.

5. Give three examples of other polymetric substances.

HIGH-FASHION POLYMER COLORS

EXPERIMENT RESULTS SHEET

Burgundy

Level 7 or 8	Level 4 or 5	Level 2 or 3

Deep Red

Level 7 or 8	Level 4 or 5	Level 2 or 3

Blue

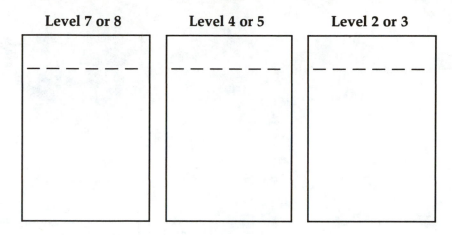

| Level 7 or 8 | Level 4 or 5 | Level 2 or 3 |

Bright Yellow

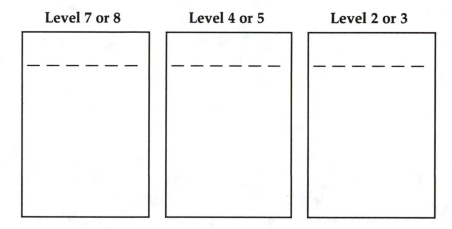

| Level 7 or 8 | Level 4 or 5 | Level 2 or 3 |

HIGH-FASHION POLYMER COLORS

REVIEW QUESTIONS

1. Describe the difference in the color results between traditional semipermanent colors and the polymers.

2. Can polymer colors be completely removed from the hair?

3. What makes polymer colors penetrate the cuticle?

4. Is use of these high-fashion polymers recommended on gray hair?

5. Are polymers compatible with permanent waving?

EFFECTS OF ARTIFICIAL HEAT ON POLYMER COLORS

EXPERIMENT RESULTS SHEET

Light Polymer Color

**10 Minutes
Warm Dryer**   **30 Minutes
Hot Dryer**

Color Name and Number _____

Manufacturer _____

Dark Polymer Color

**10 Minutes
Warm Dryer**   **30 Minutes
Hot Dryer**

Color Name and Number _____

Manufacturer _____

THE EFFECTS OF ARTIFICIAL HEAT ON POLYMER COLORS

REVIEW QUESTIONS

1. Were the color differences significant between the swatches processed with less time and heat and those processed with the greater time and heat?

2. Which method of processing creates a semipermanent color?

3. Which method of processing creates a permanent color?

4. Is a predisposition test required before use of a polymer color?

   Why?

5. Why are the colors achieved with the polymer colors so vivid?

PURE VEGETABLE HENNA

EXPERIMENT RESULTS SHEET

Level 5 or 6   **Level 3 or 4**   **Level 1 or 2**

Product _____

Formulation _____

Timing _____

Comments _____

_____

PURE VEGETABLE HENNA

REVIEW QUESTIONS

1. To which classification does pure henna belong?

2. Describe the physical and chemical changes that occur in the hair shaft when it is colored with henna.

3. Under what pH range does henna work most efficiently?

4. Is the use of pure henna recommended on gray hair?

5. How does pure henna interfere with permanent waving?

PURE HENNA WITH ORGANIC ADDITIVES

EXPERIMENT RESULTS SHEET

Beet Juice

Vinegar and Lemon Juice

Allspice

Cinnamon

Nutmeg

Paprika

PURE HENNA WITH ORGANIC ADDITIVES

REVIEW QUESTIONS

1. Did the additives make a noticeable change in the color?

   How would you alter the formulas?

2. Is the addition of H_2O_2 to henna recommended?

3. Describe two advantages of using henna rather than aniline derivative tints.

4. Describe two disadvantages of using henna rather than aniline derivative tints.

5. What is a Henna Reng?

TESTING FOR METALLIC DEPOSITS ON THE HAIR SHAFT

EXPERIMENT RESULTS SHEET

Metallic Colorings Used on Swatches:

1.   2.

3.   4.

5.   6.

7.   8.

Comments _____

_____

METALLIC DYES

REVIEW QUESTIONS

1. What descriptive terms used by manufacturers indicate that the coloring product is a metallic hair dye

2. What type of color selection is available with metallic hair dyes?

3. Describe the chemical and physical action of metallic hair dyes..

4. Why are metallic hair dyes not used professionally?

5. How would you proceed with your client consultation and color service if you suspected prior use of metallic hair dyes?

LEVEL 1—BLACK TINT COMPARISON

EXPERIMENT RESULTS SHEET

Level 2
Dark Brown

Level 4
Light Brown

Level 6
Dark Blonde

Level 8
Light Blonde

Color Name and Number _____

Manufacturer _____

Formula _____

Timing _____

Comments _____

LEVEL 1—BLACK TINT COMPARISON

REVIEW QUESTIONS

1. Compare the color results on the different natural color levels.

2. Did this tint do more lifting or depositing?

3. List five safety precautions to exercise when handling oxidation tints.

4. List five other names commercially used for oxidation tints.

5. Describe the chemical and physical changes that occur within the hair shaft as the color processes.

LEVEL 3—MEDIUM BROWN TINT COMPARISON

EXPERIMENT RESULTS SHEET

Level 2
Dark Brown

Level 4
Light Brown

Level 6
Dark Blonde

Level 8
Light Blonde

Color Name and Number _____

Manufacturer _____

Formula _____

Timing _____

Comments _____

LEVEL 3—MEDIUM BROWN TINT COMPARISON

REVIEW QUESTIONS

1. Compare the color results on the different natural color levels.

2. Did this tint do more lifting or depositing?

3. What type of dyes are used in oxidation tints?

4. List three suspected health hazards of using oxidation tints.

5. What is the purpose of adding protein to oxidation tints?

LEVEL 7—MEDIUM BLONDE TINT COMPARISON

EXPERIMENT RESULTS SHEET

Level 2
Dark Brown

Level 4
Light Brown

Level 6
Dark Blonde

Level 8
Light Blonde

Color Name and Number _____

Manufacturer _____

Formula _____

Timing _____

Comments _____

LEVEL 7—MEDIUM BLONDE TINT COMPARISON

REVIEW QUESTIONS

1. Compare the color results on the different natural color levels.

2. Did this tint do more lifting or depositing?

3. Is a predisposition test necessary before giving an oxidation tint?

4. Can this product be used over a metallic dye?

5. Is paraphenylenediamine found in all oxidation tints?

LEVEL 10—LIGHTEST BLONDE TINT COMPARISON

EXPERIMENT RESULTS SHEET

**Level 2
Dark Brown**

**Level 4
Light Brown**

**Level 6
Dark Blonde**

**Level 8
Light Blonde**

Color Name and Number _____

Manufacturer _____

Formula _____

Timing _____

Comments _____

LEVEL 10—LIGHTEST BLONDE TINT COMPARISON

REVIEW QUESTIONS

1. The formula for a high lift tint contains a smaller percentage of _____

and a larger percentage of _____ than

traditional tints.

2. Why must an oxidation tint be applied immediately after mixing?

3. Which ingredients work to improve the resulting condition of the hair after a tint?

4. Explain why the term tint is used in client consultation rather than dye.

5. What is the difference between the base and the coupler?

LEVEL 10—BLONDE TINT
FORMULATED WITH HIGH AND LOW VOLUME H₂O₂

EXPERIMENT RESULTS SHEET

10 Volume

20 Volume

30 Volume

40 Volume

Color Name and Number _____

Manufacturer _____

Formulation _____

Timing _____

Comments _____

LEVEL 10—BLONDE TINT FORMULATED WITH HIGH AND LOW VOLUME H₂O₂

REVIEW QUESTIONS

1. Describe the color differences between the swatches tinted with the four different volumes of hydrogen peroxide.

2. Name the three types of hydrogen peroxide.

3. List four uses for hydrogen peroxide outside the beauty industry.

4. Is hydrogen peroxide a natural or manmade product?

5. Describe how the compound changes when the lid is left off a bottle of hydrogen peroxide.

LEVEL 5—AUBURN TINT FORMULATED WITH HIGH AND LOW VOLUME H$_2$O$_2$

EXPERIMENT RESULTS SHEET

10 Volume   **20 Volume**

30 Volume   **40 Volume**

Color Name and Number _____

Manufacturer _____

Formulation _____

Timing _____

Comments _____

LEVEL 5—AUBURN TINT FORMULATED WITH HIGH AND LOW VOLUME H$_2$O$_2$

REVIEW QUESTIONS

1. Describe the color differences between the swatches tinted with the four different volumes of hydrogen peroxide.

2. What does a "pop" indicate when opening a bottle of hydrogen peroxide?

3. What is the pH of pure hydrogen peroxide?

   What is the pH range of hydrogen peroxide produced for the cosmetology industry?

4. List three important considerations in safely storing hydrogen peroxide.

5. How long should properly cared for hydrogen peroxide remain stable and potent?

LEVEL 3—BROWN TINT FORMULATED WITH HIGH AND LOW VOLUME H_2O_2

EXPERIMENT RESULTS SHEET

10 Volume

20 Volume

30 Volume

40 Volume

Color Name and Number _____

Manufacturer _____

Formulation _____

Timing _____

Comments _____

_____

LEVEL 3—BROWN TINT FORMULATED WITH HIGH AND LOW VOLUME H_2O_2

REVIEW QUESTIONS

1. Describe the color differences between the swatches tinted with the four different volumes of hydrogen peroxide.

2. What is the technical name for the color molecules that create natural hair color?

3. Describe how diffusion of pigment creates a lighter hair color.

4. What is the technical name for melanin that has been treated with a hydrogen peroxide solution?

5. List three advantages of both cream and liquid peroxide.

WHITE AND SILVER TONING WITH FILLERS

EXPERIMENT RESULTS SHEET

White Toner		Silver Toner	
With Filler	**Without Filler**	**With Filler**	**Without Filler**

Filler Name and Manufacturer _____

Tint Name and Manufacturer_____

Tint Formula _____

Method Used _____

Timing _____

Comments _____

WHITE AND SILVER TONING WITH FILLERS

REVIEW QUESTIONS

1. Describe the color difference between the swatches treated and not treated with filler.

2. Why was the filler dried into the hair before color application?

3. What difference would have occurred in the color if a different method of filler application had been used?

4. Name the two basic classifications of fillers.

5. What are the two main purposes of fillers?

BLONDE TINTING WITH FILLERS

EXPERIMENT RESULTS SHEET

Warm Blonde

With Filler	Without Filler

Neutral Blonde

With Filler	Without Filler

Ash Blonde

With Filler	Without Filler

Filler Name and Manufacturer _____

Tint Name and Manufacturer _____

Tint Formula _____

Method Used _____

Timing _____

Comments _____

BLONDE TINTING WITH FILLERS

REVIEW QUESTIONS

1. Describe the color differences between the swatches treated and not treated with filler.

2. What type of color correction and porosity control is achieved with this type of application?

3. Are all fillers "protein fillers"?

4. Describe three hair coloring problems that might be solved by the use of a filler.

5. How do you test the hue, intensity, and depth of a filler before formulation?

BROWN TINTING WITH FILLERS

EXPERIMENT RESULTS SHEET

Light Brown

With Filler   **Without Filler**

Medium Brown

With Filler   **Without Filler**

Dark Brown

With Filler   **Without Filler**

Filler Name and Manufacturer _____

Tint Name and Manufacturer _____

Tint Formula _____

Method Used _____

Timing _____

Comments _____

BROWN TINTING WITH FILLERS

REVIEW QUESTIONS

1. Describe the color differences between the swatches treated and not treated with filler.

2. What type of color correction and porosity control is achieved with this type of application?

3. Describe in detail how you would use the Artist's Concept of the Laws of Color to correct a tint formulation that created green tones in brown hair.

4. What is the average pH of both classifications of fillers?

5. How safe are fillers for consumer use?

REFRESHING TINTED RED HAIR WITH FILLERS

EXPERIMENT RESULTS SHEET

Light Red	Medium Red	Burgundy Red

Filler Name and Manufacturer _____

Conditioner Name and Manufacturer _____

Formula _____

Timing _____

Comments _____

REFRESHING TINTED RED HAIR WITH FILLERS

REVIEW QUESTIONS

1. What type of color correction and porosity control is achieved with this type of application?

2. Why is a nonpolymer conditioner recommended for this process?

3. Why is the hair shampooed before this treatment?

4. Describe three instances in which this technique could be used to solve a hair coloring problem.

5. Describe the process that causes fillers to attach to the hair shaft.

RED TINTING ON NATURAL LEVEL 2—DARK BROWN

EXPERIMENT RESULTS SHEET

Level 9

Level 7

Level 5

Level 3

Color Name and Manufacturer _____

Formula _____

Timing _____

Comments _____

RED TINTING ON NATURAL LEVEL 2—DARK BROWN

REVIEW QUESTIONS

1. What is the average sulfur content of hair?

2. What is the average sulfur content of red hair?

3. What effect does this have on coloring naturally red hair?

4. What factors lead to confusion when giving clients information about red hair?

RED TINTING ON NATURAL LEVEL 5—LIGHTEST BROWN

EXPERIMENT RESULTS SHEET

Level 9

Level 7

Level 5

Level 3

Color Name and Manufacturer _____

Formula _____

Timing _____

Comments _____

RED TINTING ON NATURAL LEVEL 5—LIGHTEST BROWN

REVIEW QUESTIONS

1. How does the sun cause excessive brassiness in red hair?

2. How does color fadeage cause excessive brassiness?

3. How can excessive brassiness be prevented?

4. How and when is protein used to prevent brassiness?

5. What is the theory behind using low volume peroxides with red tints?

RED TINTING ON NATURAL LEVEL 8—LIGHT BLONDE

EXPERIMENT RESULTS SHEET

Level 9 **Level 7**

Level 5 **Level 3**

Color Name and Manufacturer _____

Formula _____

Timing _____

Comments _____

RED TINTING ON NATURAL LEVEL 8—LIGHT BLONDE

REVIEW QUESTIONS

1. How can excessive brassiness be treated with temporary color?

2. What are the pros and cons of using a soap cap to adjust the tone of the hair?

3. Can all semipermanent colors be used in conjunction with tinted auburn hair?

4. Are fillers generally used to adjust tone on natural red hair?

   Why or why not?

5. Why does the use of low volume peroxide help the burgundy reds stay on-tone?

TINT BACK TO NATURAL LEVEL 6—DARK BLONDE ON BLEACHED HAIR

EXPERIMENT RESULTS SHEET

Level 6—Dark Ash Blonde

20 Volume H_2O_2	10 Volume H_2O_2	With Filler

Level 6—Dark Warm Blonde

20 Volume H_2O_2	10 Volume H_2O_2	With Filler

Filler Name and Manufacturer _____

Tint Name and Manufacturer _____

Timing _____

Comments _____

TINT BACK TO NATURAL LEVEL 6—DARK BLONDE ON BLEACHED HAIR

REVIEW QUESTIONS

1. Describe the color differences between the swatches tinted with warm blonde and the ash blonde shades.

2. Describe the color difference between the swatches tinted with different working strengths.

3. Why is a tint back to natural so complex?

4. How can the Artist's Concept of the Law of Color be implemented to prevent unwanted tones?

5. In what instances is a tint back to natural given?

TINT BACK TO NATURAL 4—MEDIUM BROWN ON BLEACHED HAIR

EXPERIMENT RESULTS SHEET

Level 4—Medium Ash Brown

20 Volume H_2O_2	10 Volume H_2O_2	With Filler

Level 4—Medium Warm Brown

20 Volume H_2O_2	10 Volume H_2O_2	With Filler

Filler Name and Manufacturer _____

Tint Name and Manufacturer _____

Timing_____

Comments _____

TINT BACK TO NATURAL 4—MEDIUM BROWN ON BLEACHED HAIR

REVIEW QUESTIONS

1. Describe the color differences between the swatches tinted with the warm brown and the ash brown shades.

2. Describe the color difference between the swatches tinted with the different working strengths.

3. What reasons does this book give for why a client might want a tint back to natural?

   What other examples can you give from your own personal experience?

4. Why is it necessary to perform a test strand before giving a tint back to natural service?

5. What unwanted tone is most common when brown is the desired shade of the tint back to natural service?

TINT BACK TO NATURAL LEVEL 2—DARK BROWN ON BLEACHED HAIR

EXPERIMENT RESULTS SHEET

Level 2—Dark Ash Brown

20 Volume H_2O_2	10 Volume H_2O_2	With Filler

Level 2—Dark Warm Brown

20 Volume H_2O_2	10 Volume H_2O_2	With Filler

Filler Name and Manufacturer _____

Tint Name and Manufacturer _____

Timing_____

Comments _____

TINT BACK TO NATURAL LEVEL 2—DARK BROWN ON BLEACHED HAIR

REVIEW QUESTIONS

1. Describe the color differences between the swatches tinted with the dark-warm brown and the dark-ash brown shades.

2. Describe the color difference between the swatches tinted with the different working strengths.

3. Which classification of color is used for a tint back to natural?

   Why?

4. Is a predisposition test necessary before a tint back to natural?

   Why?

5. What is the purpose of using low volume hydrogen peroxide when tinting back to natural?

TONAL SELECTION FOR TINTING NON-PIGMENTED HAIR

EXPERIMENT RESULTS SHEET

Warm Tones

Gold Base	Orange Base	Red Base
– – – – –	– – – – –	– – – – –

Cool Tones

Blue Base	Green Base	Violet Base
– – – – –	– – – – –	– – – – –

Manufacturer _____

Level Used _____

Formulas:

Gold Base _____

Orange Base _____

Red Base _____

Blue Base _____

Green Base _____

Violet Base _____

TONAL SELECTION FOR TINTING NON-PIGMENTED HAIR

REVIEW QUESTIONS

1. Describe the color results of each tone.

   Gold—

   Orange—

   Red—

   Blue—

   Green—

   Violet—

2. Which bases created a tone that would probably be desired by most clients?

3. Which bases would be effective to neutralize yellowed gray hair?

4. How would you cool the results of any of these tints?

5. How would you warm the results of any of these tints?

LEVEL SELECTION FOR TINTING NON-PIGMENTED HAIR

EXPERIMENT RESULTS SHEET

Level 10
Lightest Blonde

Level 8
Light Blonde

Level 6
Dark Blonde

Level 4
Light Brown

Level 2
Dark Brown

Manufacturer _____

Formulas:

Level 10 _____

Level 8 _____

Level 6 _____

Level 4 _____

Level 2 _____

LEVEL SELECTION FOR TINTING NON-PIGMENTED HAIR

REVIEW QUESTIONS

1. Name the technical term for non-pigmented hair and give the two main classifications.

2. Compare the structure of pigmented hair to non-pigmented hair.

3. Which level of color gave the least coverage?

   Why is there a lack of coverage with this tint?

4. Which level of color gave the best coverage?

   Why did this color develop so well?

5. Which level of color turned too dark?

   Why is it too dark for the average client requesting this service?

HYDROGEN PEROXIDE VOLUME COMPARISON

EXPERIMENT RESULTS SHEET

10 Volume H$_2$O$_2$ **20 Volume H$_2$O$_2$**

30 Volume H$_2$O$_2$ **40 Volume H$_2$O$_2$**

Tint Name _____

Formula _____

Manufacturer _____

HYDROGEN PEROXIDE VOLUME COMPARISON

REVIEW QUESTIONS

1. What volume of hydrogen peroxide is generally recommended by the manufacturer for tinting gray hair?

2. What may result from the use of low volume peroxide?

3. What may result from the use of high volume peroxide?

4. List four methods of achieving the desired tone and level on salt-and-pepper hair.

5. Is 20 volume *cream* peroxide always effective on non-pigmented hair?

   Why/why not?

PRESOFTENING COMPARISON

EXPERIMENT RESULTS SHEET

Liquid Presoftener   **Oil Bleach**

Gold Based Tint   **Cream Bleach**

Formulas:

Liquid Presoftener _____

Oil Bleach _____

Gold Based Tint _____

Cream Bleach _____

PRESOFTENING COMPARISON

REVIEW QUESTIONS

1. Name the two types of presofteners.

2. On what type of hair is the presoftening service done?

3. What steps should be taken to insure proper development before resorting to presoftening?

4. Which type of presoftener do you prefer?

   Why?

5. Why is the activator not included in the formulation when using cream bleach?

TINTING PRESOFTENED HAIR

EXPERIMENT RESULTS SHEET

White or Gray Hair Swatches

Liquid	Oil Bleach	Cream Bleach	Tint

Salt and Pepper Hair Swatches

Liquid	Oil Bleach	Cream Bleach	Tint

Liquid Presoftener Formula _____

Oil Bleach Formula _____

Cream Bleach Formula _____

Tint Formula _____

Timing _____

TINTING PRESOFTENED HAIR

REVIEW QUESTIONS

1. Compare the color results of the gray or white swatches processed with the four different presofteners.

2. Compare the color results of the salt and pepper swatches processed with the four different presofteners.

3. Which presoftener is most economical to use?

4. Which presoftener is easiest to use?

   Why?

5. Which presoftener gave the best results?

KINETIC MOLECULAR THEORY

REVIEW QUESTIONS

1. In your own words, explain the Kinetic Molecular Theory.

2. Define diffusion.

3. How does bleach affect the kinetic action of the compounds in the lightening formula?

4. How does bleach affect the kinetic action normally occurring within the hair shaft?

THREE CLASSIFICATIONS OF BLEACHES

EXPERIMENT RESULTS SHEET

Oil Bleach	Cream Bleach	Powder Bleach

Name of Bleach   _____   _____   _____

Manufacturer   _____   _____   _____

Formulas   _____   _____   _____

   _____   _____   _____

   _____   _____   _____

THREE CLASSIFICATIONS OF BLEACHES

REVIEW QUESTIONS

1. Which bleaches are safe to use on the scalp?

2. What is the correct oil bleach formula for one application?

3. What is the correct cream bleach formula for one application?

4. What is the correct powder bleach formula for one application?

5. Describe the consistency of correctly mixed powder bleach.

6. What is the maximum time a lightener can be applied to the scalp?

7. Is it necessary to give a predisposition test before the application of bleach?

SEVEN STAGES OF LIGHTENING

EXPERIMENT RESULTS SHEET

Black   **Brown**   **Red**   **Red-Gold**

Gold   **Yellow**   **Pale Yellow**

Name of Bleach _____

Manufacturer _____

Formula _____

SEVEN STAGES OF LIGHTENING

REVIEW QUESTIONS

1. What are the Seven Stages of Lightening?

2. What other changes occur in the hair shaft as the color is lightened?

3. Which characteristic of the hair is the most important to observe during processing?

   Why?

4. Why do professional colorists never lighten the hair to pure white?

5. How can white blonde safely be achieved?

ACTIVATOR COMPARISON

EXPERIMENT RESULTS SHEET

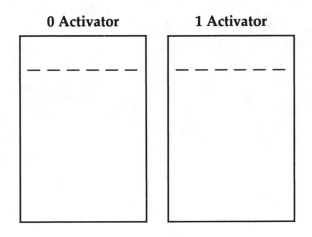

0 Activator   **1 Activator**

2 Activators   **3 Activators**   **4 Activators**

Bleach Classification _____

Name of Bleach _____

Manufacturer _____

ACTIVATOR COMPARISON

REVIEW QUESTIONS

1. Why are activators added to cream bleaches?

2. Describe the specific uses for each formulation:

   0 activator—

   1 activator—

   2 activators—

   3 activators—

   4 activators—

3. Which formulation is never used on the scalp?

EFFECTS OF ARTIFICIAL HEAT ON BLEACH

EXPERIMENT RESULTS SHEET

Oil Bleach

No Heat   **Heat**

Cream Bleach   **Powder Bleach**

No Heat   **Heat**   **No Heat**   **Heat**

Name of Bleaches _____

Manufacturers _____

Formulas _____

EFFECTS OF ARTIFICIAL HEAT ON BLEACH

REVIEW QUESTIONS

1. What differences in color, texture, and condition are evident on the 2 swatches treated with oil bleach?

2. What differences in color, texture, and condition are evident on the 2 swatches treated with cream bleach?

3. What differences in color, texture, and condition are evident on the 2 swatches treated with powder bleach?

4. In what instances is it safe to put bleach under artificial heat?

5. Which type of bleach achieved the palest level of lightening?

TONING HAIR PRE-LIGHTENED TO STAGE 5

EXPERIMENT RESULTS SHEET

Reddish Blonde Toner

10 Volume	20 Volume

Dark Ash Blonde Toner

10 Volume	20 Volume

Neutral Toner

10 Volume	20 Volume

Toner Name and Manufacturer _____

Toner Formulas _____

Timing _____

Comments _____

TONING HAIR PRE-LIGHTENED TO STAGE 5

REVIEW QUESTIONS

1. Describe the color difference between the shades achieved with 10 volume and 20 volume hydrogen peroxide.

2. How would the colors differ if the hair had been lightened to a stage 6 or 7?

3. How would the colors differ if the hair had been lightened to a stage 4?

4. What would the color results be if the hair had been bleached to pure white?

5. Why are toners not recommended for virgin color applications?

TONING HAIR PRE-LIGHTENED TO STAGE 6

EXPERIMENT RESULTS SHEET

Beige Toner

10 Volume   **20 Volume**

Ash Blonde Toner

10 Volume   **20 Volume**

Golden Blonde Toner

10 Volume   **20 Volume**

Toner Name and Manufacturer _____

Toner Formulas _____

Timing _____

Comments _____

TONING HAIR PRE-LIGHTENED TO STAGE 6

REVIEW QUESTIONS

1. Describe the color differences between the shades achieved with 10 volume and 20 volume hydrogen peroxide.

2. How would the colors differ if the hair had been lightened to a stage 7?

3. How would the colors differ if the hair had been lightened to a stage 5?

4. The amount of melanin left undiffused within the cortical layer of the hair creates the _____ for correct toning.

5. What is the main type of dye used in toners?

TONING HAIR PRE-LIGHTENED TO STAGE 7

EXPERIMENT RESULTS SHEET

White Toner

10 Volume   **20 Volume**

Silver Toner

10 Volume   **20 Volume**

Platinum Toner

10 Volume   **20 Volume**

Toner Name and Manufacturer _____

Toner Formulas _____

Timing _____

Comments _____

TONING HAIR PRE-LIGHTENED TO STAGE 7

REVIEW QUESTIONS

1. Describe the color differences between the shades achieved with 10 volume and 20 volume hydrogen peroxide.

2. What is the difference between a tint and a toner?

3. Does a toner require a predisposition test?

4. What is the significance of creating the correct foundation for toner development?

5. When pre-lightening for toner use, in addition to lightening stage foundation, what else must be created in the hair shaft for correct color development?

ACTION OF DYE SOLVENT

EXPERIMENT RESULTS SHEET

Hydrogen Peroxide Swatches

Brown   **Black**

Water Swatches

Brown   **Black**

Peroxide Formulas _____

Water Formulas _____

Brand of Dye Solvent _____

Timing _____

Comments _____

ACTION OF DYE SOLVENT

REVIEW QUESTIONS

1. When applying dye solvent to the entire head, why start where the hair is the darkest?

2. Can all dye solvents be mixed with either peroxide or water?

3. Why must the formula set a minute or two after mixing?

4. What color changes occurred in the hair swatches?

5. Describe the color differences in the swatches treated with the water and the peroxide formulas.

6. What texture and condition changes occurred in the hair swatches?

7. What happens when you bleach tinted hair without using a dye solvent first?

TINTING AFTER DYE REMOVAL—20 VOLUME FORMULATION

EXPERIMENT RESULTS SHEET

**Level 8
Light Blonde**

**Level 6
Dark Blonde**

**Level 4
Light Brown**

**Level 2
Dark Brown**

Tint Name and Manufacturer _____

Formula _____

Timing _____

Comments _____

TINTING AFTER DYE REMOVAL—20 VOLUME FORMULATION

REVIEW QUESTIONS

1. Compare the color results of your hair swatches to the color chart from which the tints were selected. Did the colors process as expected?

2. What considerations must be made when selecting a tint for application to hair previously treated with a dye solvent?

3. If the reapplication of tint processes too dark, can the dye solvent be successfully applied again?

4. Why is it advisable not to sniff dye solvent?

5. What special treatments would you recommend for the client who has received a dye solvent treatment?

TINTING AFTER DYE REMOVAL—10 VOLUME FORMULATION

EXPERIMENT RESULTS SHEET

**Level 8
Light Blonde**

**Level 6
Dark Blonde**

**Level 4
Light Brown**

**Level 2
Dark Brown**

Tint Name and Manufacturer _____

Formula _____

Timing _____

Comments _____

TINTING AFTER DYE REMOVAL—10 VOLUME FORMULATION

REVIEW QUESTIONS

1. Compare the color results of your hair swatches to the color chart from which the tints were selected. Did the colors process as expected?

2. What would have made the results more satisfactory?

3. Will this new color be truly permanent?

   Why or why not?

4. What is the purpose of using 10 volume hydrogen peroxide when tinting after using a dye solvent?

5. How does the condition and color of these swatches compare to the ones tinted with 20 volume hydrogen peroxide?

TINTING AFTER DYE REMOVAL—FILLER FORMULATION

EXPERIMENT RESULTS SHEET

Level 8
Light Blonde

Level 6
Dark Blonde

Level 4
Light Brown

Level 2
Dark Brown

Tint Name and Manufacturer _____

Formula _____

Timing _____

Comments _____

TINTING AFTER DYE REMOVAL—FILLER FORMULATION

REVIEW QUESTIONS

1. Compare the color results of your hair swatches to the color chart from which the tints were selected. Did the colors process as expected?

2. What would have made the results more satisfactory?

3. What is the purpose of using filler in the tint formula applied after use of a dye solvent?

4. Compare the condition and color results of these swatches to the ones tinted with no filler.

5. Which application procedure is used to tint the hair after a dye solvent treatment?